"Bravo, *Intuitive Eating for Life*! I wholeheartedly
freedom available to us when we embrace the presen
only to celebrate each and every meal before us, but
ment our souls receive as well."

—**Emme**, mother, model, social disrupter, coauthor of *Chicken Soup
for the Soul: Curvy and Confident*, and founder of www.truebeauty
foundation.org

"What a gift to have a book that complements *Intuitive Eating*, while also bringing meaning to why mindfulness and intuitive eating are so interconnected.
Jenna Hollenstein takes intuitive eating from its self-care framework and weaves
it into a practice that is sustained through a dedication to mindfulness, acceptance, and self-compassion. Through thought-provoking questions and exercises, she guides the reader down a path that brings unconscious perceptions
into conscious awareness, ultimately leading to decreased stress and increased
well-being. This book is a gem!"

—**Elyse Resch, MS, RDN, CEDS-S**, nutrition therapist, coauthor of
Intuitive Eating, and author of *The Intuitive Eating Workbook for Teens*

"In *Intuitive Eating for Life*, Jenna Hollenstein artfully and compassionately
bridges the gap between mindful eating and intuitive eating. If you've tried
intuitive eating and had trouble implementing the principles, this book may be
just what you are missing! It's more than a book about changing your relationship with food—it's about changing your relationship with yourself, and may
impact your life in ways that you never expected."

—**Alexis Conason, PsyD**, psychologist, and author of
The Diet-Free Revolution

"Reading *Intuitive Eating for Life* is like spending time with a trusted friend who
walks alongside you in your own journey. This book recognizes the differences
we all bring to our eating, and asks us to celebrate them instead of push against
them as diet culture has demanded of us. With sensitivity and compassion,
Jenna invites everyone to the table in this thoughtful, practical text."

—**Colleen Clemens, PhD**, director of women's, gender,
and sexuality studies at Kutztown University; and coeditor
of *Philadelphia Reflections*

"Intuitive eating often makes sense intellectually, but many people (understandably) struggle with the discomfort and uncertainty that go along with putting it into practice. With *Intuitive Eating for Life*, Hollenstein shows us how mindfulness is an essential skill that will help you 'sit with' these challenges. Full of reflection prompts, tools, and practices, this book will help you explore your relationship to food, eating, and your body from a place of compassion and curiosity."

—**Alissa Rumsey, MS, RD**, author of *Unapologetic Eating*

"Intuitive eating should be easy and straightforward—right? Often, this is not the case. Yet, we shouldn't give up on intuitive eating, as it enhances well-being. Instead, we need practices that support it. You'll find this support within Hollenstein's book. Stocked with mindfulness practices and information, this brilliant book will help deepen and sustain your intuitive eating path and build trust and confidence in your body."

—**Tracy Tylka, PhD**, professor of psychology at The Ohio State University, Intuitive Eating Scale developer, and editor of *Body Image*

"Relatable, practical, and filled with honesty, *Intuitive Eating for Life* enlists powerful mindfulness techniques to help us think about the way we approach food from an intuitive and nonrestrictive place. The 'mindful moments' sprinkled throughout the book help you tangibly find ways to apply these techniques to your everyday life without feeling overwhelmed!"

—**Bethany C. Meyers**, founder and CEO of the be.come project, and advocate for body neutrality

"I wish this book were a standard-issue user manual for having a human body! Have you tried intuitive eating and needed 'something' to make it work? *Intuitive Eating for Life* is your magic ingredient. Jenna tackles tender realities of living in a body with the gentleness and precision of a true mindfulness master, and offers a path to the cessation of suffering that arises from diet culture. Brilliant and invaluable!"

—**Erica Mather, MA**, yoga therapist; and author of *Your Body, Your Best Friend*

Intuitive Eating

How Mindfulness Can Deepen and
Sustain Your Intuitive Eating Practice

for Life

Jenna Hollenstein, MS, RD, CDN

New Harbinger Publications, Inc.

Publisher's Note

This publication is designed to provide accurate and authoritative information in regard to the subject matter covered. It is sold with the understanding that the publisher is not engaged in rendering psychological, financial, legal, or other professional services. If expert assistance or counseling is needed, the services of a competent professional should be sought.

NEW HARBINGER PUBLICATIONS is a registered trademark of New Harbinger Publications, Inc.

New Harbinger Publications is an employee-owned company.

Cover design by Sara Christian; Acquired by Ryan Buresh; Edited by Karen Levy

---

Library of Congress Cataloging-in-Publication Data

Names: Hollenstein, Jenna, author.
Title: Intuitive eating for life : how mindfulness can deepen and sustain your intuitive eating practice / Jenna Hollenstein, MS, RDN, CDN.
Description: Oakland, CA : New Harbinger Publications, [2022] | Includes bibliographical references.
Identifiers: LCCN 2022028037 | ISBN 9781684039401 (trade paperback)
Subjects: LCSH: Diet--Psychological aspects--Popular works. | Mindfulness (Psychology)--Popular works. | Body image--Popular works. | BISAC: SELF-HELP / Eating Disorders & Body Image | BODY, MIND & SPIRIT / Mindfulness & Meditation
Classification: LCC RM222 .H65 2022 | DDC 613.2--dc23/eng/20220713
LC record available at https://lccn.loc.gov/2022028037

Printed in the United States of America

24   23   22

10   9   8   7   6   5   4   3   2   1   First Printing

This book is dedicated to your intelligent body, compassionate heart, and flexible mind. May you embody your true brilliance.

Contents

PART IV: Mindfulness of Phenomena

Introduction

Welcome to the first page of the rest of your life. That might sound dramatic but I mean it—this is life-changing stuff. I'm glad you're here.

You've probably already heard of Intuitive Eating. It's everywhere and people are talking about how great it is. Perhaps you bought the *Intuitive Eating* book or workbook. Felt enormous relief. Tried to let go of rigid control over how you ate. Experimented with some forbidden foods.

After decades of dieting, it's liberating to think you could eat what you love without guilt or shame. But finding a balanced approach to eating without restricting or binging feels impossible. Without the structure of rules and diets, you may have begun to feel unmoored. Without restricting, you gained weight. You felt you were losing control, confirming you can't trust your body. Perhaps you concluded there was something different about your body and that Intuitive Eating won't work for you.

Know you're not alone. Intuitive Eating—the evidence-based model created by registered dietitians Evelyn Tribole and Elyse Resch that will completely transform your relationship with food and body—is simple but not easy to do. Especially on your own.

Intuitive Eating is not the "eat when you're hungry, stop when you're full" diet. It does not progress linearly through neatly organized principles. It unfolds differently for each person doing it, so while there are some common milestones, individual variations in experience can feel unexpected and insurmountable.

Many people have found success with Intuitive Eating by working with a professional like myself, a nutrition therapist trained by its creators. Someone to reflect your experience back to you—encouraging you to celebrate your progress, guiding your attention, recognizing obstacles, and supporting your work to deepen self-knowledge. Simply being in relationship with someone who holds space for you and believes in you can help you sustain Intuitive Eating when things inevitably become difficult.

This book is not meant to replace the support of a Certified Intuitive Eating Counselor, which, if accessible, is always recommended. Unfortunately, this professional help is not equitably available. It is expensive and time consuming. It's not easy to find a clinician who gets you, looks like you, understands what it's like to live in your body. And it is often not of long enough duration to support the lifelong unfolding of Intuitive Eating. Becoming an Intuitive Eater involves uncertainty and discomfort, two things you might not feel well equipped to deal with. There's no manual explaining how to get comfortable with discomfort. Given the varying experiences with Intuitive Eating, its inherent challenges, and the need for healing through relationship, where does that leave you?

This is where mindfulness comes in.

Mindfulness Bridges the Gap

Mindfulness trains you to stay with yourself, even (or especially) when things get uncomfortable. Mindfulness is a way of life in which you place attention on your moment-to-moment reality. You notice and tend to bodily sensations, emotions, thoughts, and the environment with curiosity, compassion, and gentleness. You expand to tolerate the full range of your emotions and experiences—the good, the bad, and everything in between.

Mindfulness helps you recognize when you are replaying something from your past, fantasizing about the future, or simply daydreaming, and to come back to the present moment again and again. In coming back, you can recognize what is actually happening in your life—not what you fear will happen, wish would happen, or think should happen.

When you are authentically in your real life, you see yourself honestly. You recognize how you personally (and we as a society) have suffered at the hands of the diet culture and its inhumane expectations. You inventory its costs to your life. You assess the dissonance between your thoughts and actions in pursuit of thinness and your true values. You make connections between beliefs, thoughts, emotions, and actions and can course-correct in real time. This reorientation toward your genuine self lets you live with openness, purpose, and joy.

Mindfulness also connects you with your body, mind, and heart in ways that help you navigate difficulty. It strengthens resilience and cognitive flexibility so that discomfort and uncertainty don't derail you. Instead, you can soften toward them and learn what they need to teach you.

Finally, mindfulness puts you in deeper relationship with yourself and others. This enhances self-compassion and sharpens self-observation. Ultimately, you build confidence and trust in your body's self-regulation and your mind's flexibility. When you trust your body and feel confident in your basic goodness, how you relate to others is exponentially improved.

It's a hard sell to recommend getting comfortable with discomfort. But suffering is a universal human experience. It is central to why you struggle with food and your body. It is also how you will ultimately heal.

As you move through the book, you will notice many moments of uncertainty and discomfort. You will see how they reveal important information about your relationship with food and body—and likely your relationship with life in general—and present opportunities to transform confusion into wisdom and compassion. There are paradoxes inherent in this work: you are capable of authentic change, but the responsibility does not rest solely on you; you can make changes on an individual level, but your body, all bodies, are part of something larger.

What Is Mindfulness and Where Does It Come From?

Mindfulness comes from ancient Buddhist teachings about the nature of reality. The first teaching given by the Buddha once he attained enlightenment—the four noble truths—is the closest you'll ever get to that elusive manual on how to get comfortable with discomfort.

The four noble truths—those nonnegotiable qualities of life in a human body—are:

1. The truth of suffering

2. The cause of suffering

3. The cessation of suffering

4. The path to the cessation of suffering

The first noble truth does not mean life is terrible. It means we all experience some *dis*-ease in our lives. Sickness, old age, and death are examples, but so are the icky feeling of a too-tight waistband and the disappointment of bad takeout.

The second noble truth is suffering is caused by resistance to the first noble truth. When we fight the truth of suffering and desperately try to only experience pleasure, we end up miserable. The third noble truth is that there is a way out, while the fourth noble truth defines the path, which includes right understanding, right thought, right speech, right action, right livelihood, right effort, right mindfulness, and right concentration.

Mindfulness is essential in the fourth noble truth, the path to the cessation of suffering. It is infused into every other part of the path. Its most basic meaning is to be fully in the moment. Mindfulness teaches you to recognize each moment as sacred and as yet unexperienced. Throughout this book, you will see how certain moments of your life reveal important information about your relationship with food and body—if you pay attention to them. By noticing these poignant moments, naming them, and working with them as they are, you will ultimately transform that relationship.

The Four Noble Truths of Having a Body

My clients always hear me say, "Don't leave out your body!" The word "mindfulness" is a misnomer because of its emphasis on mind. In reality, what happens in the body is even more important. When the mind recognizes and interprets what is happening in the physical and emotional body as it interacts with itself, with others, and with its environment, awareness happens.

In the spirit of not leaving out the body, let's apply the four noble truths to the body and how they relate to food, eating, and dieting:

1. Existing in the world in a human body is hard.

2. Trying to bypass this difficulty by dieting and controlling your body only increases your suffering.

3. There is a way out that includes working *with* instead of *against* your body.

4. The path is framed by mindfully working through the ten principles of Intuitive Eating.

Having a body is hard. It can get sick or injured. It hurts sometimes and ages day by day. Parts of your body may not work like they used to, and your body may not always perform or appear as you wish. This can be disappointing and upsetting. There is nothing you can do to change this. Without perspective, these truths can be difficult to accept.

The diet culture—the system of industries rooted in healthism and Eurocentric beauty ideals—preys on your difficulty accepting this truth. It presents weight loss as a means to relieve or avoid suffering, creating a perfect storm in which you feel obligated to "work on" your body, always trying to improve it, never letting it be enough. Diet culture creates inhumane standards to achieve "worthiness" few can attain. It invents problems and then sells you the solutions. It distracts you from what you probably value a lot more than beauty and thinness: happiness, connection, being of benefit.

You can break this cycle by reimagining your relationship with food and your body. This involves learning to work with your body: listening to it, asking it what it wants and needs, acknowledging its basic goodness. And finally learning to work with discomfort and uncertainty.

The path to the cessation of suffering with our bodies is paved by the ten principles of Intuitive Eating:

1. Reject the diet mentality

2. Honor your hunger

3. Make peace with food

4. Challenge the food police

5. Discover the satisfaction factor

6. Feel your fullness

7. Cope with your feelings with kindness

8. Respect your body

9. Movement: feel the difference

10. Honor your health: gentle nutrition

As of the fourth edition of *Intuitive Eating*, "Discover the satisfaction factor" was placed before "Feel your fullness." Principle 7 was edited to say, "Cope with your feelings with kindness" instead of "...without food." And the word "exercise" in principle 9 is now "movement." I share this because it emphasizes how we all continue to evolve in our understanding of Intuitive Eating, even its creators!

Where Intuitive Eating and Mindfulness Intersect

Intuitive Eating and mindfulness are innately compatible and complementary. Both seek to work with reality. In one sense, reality is that certain things are out of your control, while others are at least somewhat within your control. The size and shape of your body are largely determined by factors out of your control, such as genetics. How you have come to perceive your body is determined by larger systems that center thinness, whiteness, youth, and beauty. Knowing this, how you think and feel about your body is subject to your influence: you can change how you think and feel to focus less on how to change your body and more on how to care for it. Reality also means the constantly changing needs of your human body, how your body protects you from starvation (i.e., dieting), and how battling with your body only intensifies suffering. By working with reality, you stand squarely in the middle of your real life, not some imagined future where everything is perfect.

Mindfulness helps you practice the first principle of Intuitive Eating by recognizing that diets don't work. Your own lived experience reveals how you have repeated the same pattern: trying one diet after the next or committing to restrictive lifestyle changes you don't realize are diets. Once you accept this truth, there is no going back.

Intuitive Eating and mindfulness are embodied practices deeply connected with interoception—the ability to sense inward, accurately interpret what is presently happening in your body, and respond with precision and kindness. Honing interoception through mindfulness supports you to honor hunger, discover satisfaction, respect fullness, develop a sustainable movement practice, and ultimately experiment with nutrition. This work is enlivened by respect for your innate intelligence: you are the only true expert of you. You possess wisdom sharpened by working with your mind and listening to your body and heart.

Intuitive Eating and mindfulness teach you the importance of tolerating discomfort. Making peace with food, continuing to challenge the food police, and more precisely sensing and responding to emotions require you to feel, allow, and stay with your experience even as it becomes uncomfortable. This helps you recognize automatic reactions to discomfort. By slowing things down, you can respond skillfully instead of reacting automatically, gradually breaking dysfunctional cycles that cause you harm.

Mindfulness helps you recognize how Intuitive Eating affects your life in small and large ways. You learn that whatever you do, you are just trying to feel okay. Sometimes this is through dysfunctional thoughts or behaviors, but mindfulness and Intuitive Eating support you to feel okay by enacting true self-care: learning to respect your body unconditionally, cultivating self-compassion, and bravely turning toward your real life empowers you to work with each experience authentically.

Finally, both Intuitive Eating and mindfulness are paths, not destinations or endpoints. You can't mess them up. Both processes unfold at an appropriate pace for you. And—spoiler alert—this unfolding continues for the rest of your life.

How to Use This Book

This book is a complement to the *Intuitive Eating* book and *The Intuitive Eating Workbook*. It is a resource to return to as your Intuitive Eating practice evolves over your life. During physical, emotional, social, and spiritual changes, you can return to this book to stay connected with and deepen your Intuitive Eating practice.

The book is structured within the Four Foundations of Mindfulness, a Buddhist framework that increases awareness and removes obstacles to working with life on life's terms. The Four Foundations are mindfulness of body, mindfulness of feelings, mindfulness of mind (or thoughts), and mindfulness of dhammas (or phenomena). Each foundation of mindfulness is related to the others, as are the ten principles of Intuitive Eating. That interconnectedness does cause some overlap.

When you begin reading, consider going all the way through the whole book and then returning to a specific section to dig in. This is a resource for any time you encounter obstacles on your Intuitive Eating path. Consider it my way of being there with you: holding space for you, cheering you on, reminding you that you were born an Intuitive Eater, and reassuring you that the painful points teach you exactly what you need to learn. So, please stay.

"Mindful Moments" are sprinkled throughout the book. Get a journal, open a note in your phone, or start a document in which you record thoughts, feelings, reactions, and "noticings." These exercises will help you make the practice truly yours: to deepen awareness, conduct experiments, observe yourself nonjudgmentally, and continually speak to yourself with compassion.

I encourage you to celebrate progress, early and often. My definition of progress may be different from yours: it's progress when you notice yourself in the moment, having different experiences than you did before, responding in intentional ways, and connecting the dots between thoughts, feelings, and behaviors. If you don't celebrate progress with a little "p" and hold out for Progress with a big "P," you'll miss all the ways in which you are already eating intuitively.

There are also materials available for download, including supportive resources and additional meditation instructions, at the website for this book: http://www.newharbinger.com/49401. (See the very back of this book for more details.)

Before We Begin

I have written this book with the aspiration of helping you regain trust and confidence in your body, mind, and heart because I believe that will ultimately make the world a better place. I have done so from a limited position, however, so there are likely aspects of your experience that are not adequately or sensitively addressed here. For that I apologize in advance. I benefit from substantial and unearned privilege: I am a white, thin, able-bodied, educated, middle-class woman. I have one child, a babysitter, and child-care support from my parents, without whom none of this would be possible. My partner works full time, which has allowed me to write a book. I live with depression and anxiety (common mental illnesses I feel compelled to destigmatize) and chronic pain. I have had the privilege of learning to meditate and to study the dharma. This has changed everything for me.

While this book speaks to you as an individual, which suggests that accepting your body is a personal responsibility, the truth is that there are unjust and inhumane social systems that make us feel not at home in our bodies. How to change those systems is beyond the scope of this book but has been addressed well by many wonderful authors, social justice warriors, and activists. Please explore some of these other titles in the resources offered online at http://www.newharbinger.com/49401.

With this understanding between us, let's set out on the path of applying mindfulness to Intuitive Eating.

CHAPTER 1

Mindfulness Is a Form of Self-Care and Respect

Whether you feel grateful for a full life or long to fill haunting gaps, there is likely a missing piece that you can't quite find: how to get your food in order and your body under control. That missing piece is so essential it means you can't complete the rest of the puzzle.

Your body might cause you great suffering. Perhaps you experience discrimination based on your body at work, in relationships, at the doctor's office. Shopping for clothing is painful and embarrassing. Going to the movies, sitting on a plane, riding a roller coaster—none of these spaces were made for you. So you focus on becoming smaller: suffer now through diet after diet, so that you experience comfort, inclusion, and visibility later.

You "just don't feel yourself" at this weight. You know diets don't work but wonder if you could just find the right one. You have tried to let go, but you simply cannot rest until your body is smaller, more toned, and less (#Roxane Gay) unruly.

Unfortunately, you are not the first to think or feel any of these ways. Our sick culture places an inordinate amount of value on appearance, specifically thinness, youth, and beauty. It tells you in subtle and not-so-subtle ways that buying the products and services that move you toward these ideals will ultimately bring you the happiness and belonging you desire.

You've been absorbing these messages since you were a child. They shaped the neural pathways your mind travels again and again, linking thinness with self-worth, fatness with danger, dieting with righteous effort, and restrained eating with discipline, health, and control. When you stick with a program, you feel worthy. When you can't, you feel like a failure.

When your body does not comply with the culture's expectations—which you have internalized and come to think of as your own—you think the problem is you.

This is how many people move through the world, though the specifics vary widely based on intersections of body size, race, class, age, ability, gender identity, sexual orientation, citizenship, geographic region, and whether you are neurodiverse. Your negative relationship with your body taints your relationship with your life, tingeing everything with a not-quite-okay-ness that needs fixing.

I used to feel this way: never good enough, never worthy of unconditional love. I was obsessed with self-improvement and ways to become better, different, ideally someone else. Dieting—though I rarely called it that—was one way I tried to change myself. Years later, I stopped drinking alcohol and saw how I used drinking, eating, and dieting to have a different experience than the one I found too painful to face. I finally saw how my intolerance for uncertainty and discomfort drove me to painful thoughts and actions that only deepened my suffering.

I felt this poorly about myself while simultaneously benefiting from the privilege of being a thin, cis, able-bodied white woman. I do not know what it feels like to live in a fat body. A black or brown body. A disabled body. A trans body. These distinctions matter. Each marginalized identity you possess exponentially increases the bias that you suffer. You might internalize and weaponize these biases against yourself. The basic message is this: wanting to be other than you are is painful. But depending on their personal experience, people have varying and more complex reasons for wanting to be different.

A year into recovery from alcoholism, I meditated for the first time. As I continued to practice and study Buddhist teachings, I learned that they have nothing to do with self-improvement. Meditation, and the world of mindfulness that is derived from it, is about being with yourself as you are.

Mindfulness is a way of paying attention to yourself—your thoughts and feelings, your actions and reactions—that provides invaluable insights into what is really happening, what is working for you, and what is not. I have come to think of mindfulness as the most basic form of self-care, self-respect, and self-love. This is available to everyone.

Ironically, the more I meditate and study, the more I both stay the same person I always was and simultaneously evolve and change. As Carl Rogers wrote in *On Becoming a Person*, "The curious paradox is that when I accept myself just as I am, then I can change."[1]

The changes brought about through mindfulness may not be what you were hoping for. They are not the result of treating yourself as a problem to be fixed, but of learning to work with yourself as you are. This is a very different way of relating to yourself. It will take time to change the neural pathways that make you feel unworthy, that lead you to strive to be different. Yet it is possible, with patience, attention, and practice. And it can continue throughout your life.

Your Changing Brain

As mindfulness practices reached the West, scientists have studied their mechanisms and effects. Their research shows how paying attention in certain ways changes the structure and function of the brain and alters how you experience your life.[2]

Mindfulness practices like meditation increase gray matter in the parts of your brain that control decision making, and decrease matter in the parts controlling the fight, flight, or freeze response. These changes alter how you experience unpleasant states. Pain, fear, stress, anxiety, and discomfort can be felt purely and not automatically interpreted as dangerous. When you sense less danger, you can become more curious about your feelings. If your habitual reaction is to self-medicate with food or disordered behaviors, you might instead find other ways to meet your actual needs.

Mindfulness sharpens interoception, the ability to sense and accurately interpret what is happening in your body in real time.[3] Hunger, fullness, and satisfaction can be felt in the body, as can fatigue, fear, loneliness, and all your other states and emotions. When you react in damaging, habitual ways less often, you can more skillfully respond to what your body is communicating. You understand what you need and feel empowered to practice self-care. You won't practice mindfulness because of increased gray matter. But you might because of how it makes you feel and how it affects your life.

Mindfulness practices are associated with physical and mental health benefits. The stress hormone cortisol decreases.[4] Depression, anxiety, obsessive-compulsive disorder, substance use, and chronic pain are mediated.[5] Focus and concentration increase.[6] Scientists have even begun to understand meditation's famous increase in compassion.[7]

How to Pay Attention

Jon Kabat-Zinn defined mindfulness as "the awareness that arises from paying attention, on purpose, in the present moment and nonjudgmentally."[8] Most people understand mindfulness is about paying attention. What they miss is the importance of *how* to pay attention.

If you have dieted a good portion of your life, you clearly know how to pay attention—to nutrition labels, macros, calories, and every perceived microscopic change in your body. You have paid attention to thin-spiration and fit-spiration blogs and social media accounts. Paying attention is not a lacking skill for the dieter, but gentleness is.

Gentleness is implicit in allowing things to just be—including yourself. Mindfulness helps you see things clearly, honestly: as they are. Before you can judge them as positive, negative, or neutral, things just *are*.

Experiencing life in this pure, raw way can make it come alive. What was once straightforward, unexciting, and black and white suddenly becomes Technicolor, richly textured, magnetizing. At least that's how it's been for me.

Food tastes brilliant, flowers are tender and gorgeous, your love for others is deep and otherworldly. Your suffering also comes into focus. Heartbreak aches dully in your chest, anger stokes a fire in your belly, shame feels like your entire body is caving in. But with the stability gained from mindfulness, you are more able to stay with these emotions. And the staying starts to feel important. Even your suffering is rich, part of what makes you alive.

When life feels richer, you need less entertainment, less nonstop pleasure. You can be right where you are. Turning toward your in-the-moment experience is an act of true self-care. You might start to think of such moments as "near-life experiences" in which you are fully present. Waking up to your actual life is the best use of your time, energy, and effort I can imagine, and both mindfulness and Intuitive Eating support you to do this.

Paying attention with gentleness is the best way to practice body respect, which I define as continuing to treat your body with kindness and meet its most basic needs even when you don't feel good about it (or a part of it). You feed it, give it rest, and allow it to feel comfort and pleasure. It is unrealistic to expect yourself to love all parts of your body all the time. That basic self-care should be unconditional and not contingent on ever-changing, and completely normal, feelings about your body.

How the Four Foundations of Mindfulness Support Intuitive Eating

This book is framed within the Four Foundations of Mindfulness—body, feelings, thoughts, and phenomena. But what do these have to do with food, self-care, and body respect?

Mindfulness of body practices bring greater awareness to what your body is communicating—what it is feeling and what it is asking for. Your body is innately intelligent. It knows what it needs.

Mindfulness of feelings—built on the foundation of a body stabilized by unconditional caring—works with your emotions with gentleness. An intolerance for strong or negative emotions likely contributes to your confusion and suffering about your body. Seeing your emotions clearly makes it possible to identify and meet your true needs.

Mindfulness of mind, or thought, guides you to remodel your brain by choosing to think thoughts that align with gentleness and self-compassion instead of dieting thoughts that have driven you to hate yourself. You literally rewire your brain.

Mindfulness of phenomena is about making connections between the different parts of your experience. For example, if you tend to approach food with rigid control, you probably apply that to other parts of your life, such as work, family, and relationships. Healing your relationship with food and body can filter into every other part of your life. And those of others.

Irene's Story

Irene struggled with body image, particularly after menopause. It took patience, consistent nourishment, and exploration of supportive resources like podcasts, research papers (she was into that), and books before she could consider the change work that needed to be done was emotional and not physical.

First, we met her biological needs, ensuring she was getting "enough." With a body stabilized by proper physical care, she could delve into the emotional aspects of her relationship with food and body. For support, she started a body gratitude journal and discovered there was much she appreciated about her body and took for granted. Initially, this discovery provoked self-aggression and shame "for having superficial thoughts." We processed this by normalizing how she had been conditioned by the culture to do so. Gradually, Irene softened into the messiness of her experience in a human body.

A few weeks later, she caught a cold and felt a different level of self-awareness and self-care arising. By paying compassionate and mindful attention to her needs, she acknowledged her hunger and cravings for foods that were particularly soothing, such as oatmeal and chicken soup. She emerged from that illness seeing the connection between tending to her physical body, her feelings, and her thoughts. Mindfulness and Intuitive Eating paved the way.

MINDFUL MOMENT: Checking In with Yourself

As you work with this book, ask the following questions and capture any "notic-ings" in your journal. When you feel hunger, think something specific, or feel garden-variety discomfort, these questions will help you build trust and confidence in your body, mind, and heart:

- What emotions am I feeling right now?

- How comfortable do I feel working directly with these emotions?

- What sensations are present in my body in this moment?

- How confident am I in interpreting these sensations?

- What is the texture of my thoughts right now?

- What is it like to allow my mind to be as it is?

- How is my body/nervous system trying to protect me right now?

- What in my environment might be affecting me?

- What do I need?

- How do I know?

MINDFUL MOMENT: Shamatha-Vipashyana Meditation

Shamatha-vipashyana, mindfulness-awareness, is an open-eye breath awareness technique. Read through these instructions and then use the guided meditation found at http://www.newharbinger.com/49401.

Find a comfortable seat either in a chair with feet flat on the floor or on a meditation cushion, couch, or bed with legs crossed loosely in front of you. Sit up straight while respecting the natural curves of your spine. Your sitz bones (sitting bones) root down into whatever you are sitting on while the crown of your head reaches gently up toward the ceiling. The back of your body is strong while the front of your body is open and soft. Let your shoulder blades melt down your back and rest your hands palms down on the tops of your thighs. Think of your body as finding a balance of rest and effort.

Take a moment to scan the front of your body, releasing any tension you don't need to maintain this uplifted posture, for example, in the ankles, hip flexors, belly, chest, neck, and face. Your mouth is closed but not clamped shut. Your lips and teeth may be slightly parted. Your eyes are open with a gentle gaze cast down and in front of you at a distance of four to six feet. The breath comes in and goes out through your nose without any specific technique. Just breathe naturally.

Feel your body breathing. Locate for yourself where you feel the breath—whether at the tip of the nostrils, at the back of the throat, high up in the chest, or with the movements of the chest and/or belly—and place your mind's attention there. You are not counting breaths, following the breath, or observing the breath. You are *feeling* the breath.

As you feel the breath, your mind will continue to make thoughts. Allow your mind to be as it is, whether stormy or dreamy or slippery. Take a moment to notice how you can simultaneously feel your breath and remain aware of sights, sounds, sensations, and thoughts. Feeling the breath can peacefully coexist with awareness. As long as you stay connected with the feeling of breath even a little, no further action is required. Just sit and let yourself be.

At some point, inevitably a line of thought will take you away from the breath completely and you will become absorbed. You may be gone for mere moments or for minutes at a time until something recognizes you have forgotten you were meditating. When you realize you got lost, take an instant to acknowledge the thought. You can say silently to yourself "thinking." Then, release it and gently guide your attention back to the feeling of the breath. Begin again.

This is the practice. Still the body. Feel the breath. Let the mind be as it is. When you realize you have gotten lost, come back to the feeling of the breath. Take a fresh start.

It is important to distinguish between the two types of thought: thoughts that peacefully coexist with feeling the breath and those that take you away from it. In feeling the breath and allowing the mind to be as it is, you expand your tolerance for the full range of your experience. In recognizing when you've gotten lost and coming back again and again, you strengthen your capacity for staying present, for distinguishing the truth of right now from the fantasy of anything else.

Begin your practice gently and realistically. Consider starting with ten minutes a day, three days a week for two weeks and then reassessing. Decide where you will sit and what time. Use your journal to record your experience, simply writing down the date, number of minutes you practiced, and anything you noticed. After two weeks, if you were able to keep this commitment, consider whether you want to increase the number of days you are sitting, for example, Monday through Friday for the same ten minutes. Try this for another two weeks. If you were not able to keep your original commitment, don't worry! Try downshifting to five minutes a day or change the time to one that works better for you in your current schedule. Meditation is flexible and should never be used to feel badly about yourself.

Your shamatha practice will support you throughout this book and beyond. Think of your relationship with your meditation practice as any long-term relationship that will go through many phases. Consider how to maintain a connection with your meditation practice and allow it to work with your life.

We now dive into mindfulness of body. Before we do, take a moment to celebrate the effort you made to be here, to contemplate this different way of being in your body and in the world. Celebrate taking an interest in yourself just as you take an interest in the feeling of breath in meditation. Celebrate the simple yet sacred dignity in working with your mind rather than trying to change your body.

PART I

Mindfulness of Body

Mindfulness of body forms the foundation of a lifelong Intuitive Eating practice. It is the beginning, middle, and end of working with things as they are.

Invoking mindfulness of body, you respect your body as teacher—always in the present moment. You meet your body's basic needs unconditionally and with constancy of attention to what is arising in real time. You are guided by the sensations of your innately intelligent body—hunger, fullness, satisfaction, the desire to move, the need for rest.

Mindfulness of body involves eating regularly, adequately, and satisfyingly with a balance of protein, carbs, and fat. Getting adequate quantity and quality of sleep. Drinking enough (but not too much) water. Moving as your body asks to move, with joy and purpose. Resting when that is what's needed. Tending to stress in all its manifestations. Rediscovering play, intimacy, and sensuality. And connecting with people, places, and other resources that ground and regulate you.

CHAPTER 2

How Mindfulness Affects Your Body

When you practice mindfulness, paying attention to your experience with curiosity and without judgment, your body and brain change in subtle yet meaningful ways. These changes fuel an Intuitive Eating practice, as well as a life of presence and joy. Mindfulness and the practice of meditation remodel your brain, stabilize your nervous system, and deepen physical and emotional awareness. These changes form a loop that becomes more profound and layered over time.

Safety, food, water, rest, sleep, movement, connection, and stress management are the basic needs of every human body. If you are chronically underfed, sleep deprived, or in an unsafe environment, for example, it is not realistic or humane to try doing this work. Intuitive Eating and mindfulness are only possible in a body whose basic needs are met.

Remodeling Your Brain

When you begin to practice mindfulness, there are immediate and longer term effects. Short-term effects include shifts in circulating neurotransmitter. and hormone levels.[9] This enhances attention and relaxation. Many people feel less stress and more well-being. Heart rate, blood pressure, and respiration rate also come down. Over the longer term, with time and repetition, the structure and function of the brain are altered.[2] These changes include:

- Increased overall gray matter, enhancing intelligence and processing.

- Increased gray matter in the prefrontal cortex, improving memory and executive function. This brain area tends to shrink with age, but researchers have found fifty-year-old meditators have similar volume to twenty-five-year-olds.[10]

- Decreased mass in the amygdala, a part of the limbic system involved in emotions such as fear, anxiety, and aggression. This decrease improves emotional awareness and control.

- Weakened connections between the amygdala and the prefrontal cortex, decreasing reactivity so you can be more intentionally and skillfully responsive.

- Increased hippocampal mass, which allows new experiences to be recognized, remembered, and accessed later.

- Increased high-frequency gamma brain waves both when meditating and when just living your life, enabling greater panoramic awareness and bliss.

Brain changes brought about through mindfulness alter how you experience yourself, your life, and the world. Time seems to slow down. Your mind feels spacious. Awareness expands. And you notice what is happening as it happens. Real-time awareness powers your Intuitive Eating practice by increasing tolerance of discomfort and helping you think flexibly, seeing choices where previously you thought you had none.

Mira's Story

Mira started a messy and imperfect meditation practice with five to ten minutes a day, three days a week, in the mornings before work. She was doubtful so little time would really affect her self-awareness until one afternoon while working at home. After a long morning of remote meetings and mounting stress, Mira found herself enacting a familiar pattern, mindlessly walking to the kitchen to crunch on something as a distraction from how uncomfortable she felt. Except this time, she was moving in slow motion. Each step toward the kitchen was accompanied by self-inquiry: What are you feeling right now? What is going on in your body? Have you eaten enough? What do you need? It's okay to eat, but is that what you really need?

Mira realized she did need a snack, but she also needed some soothing. She took a cookie from the pantry and headed out the door for a walk before her next meeting. Walking and enjoying her cookie, Mira realized something had shifted in her capacity for self-awareness.

Stabilizing the Nervous System

The nervous system has always existed to protect you. If you learn one thing from this section, let it be this: your body is always trying to protect you, and whatever you do, no matter how seemingly dysfunctional, you are just trying to feel okay. Eating to soothe emotions. Restricting to feel in control. Exercising to compensate for overeating. Collapsing into depression when nothing is going right. All are actions you might take when your nervous system is dysregulated and trying to feel okay.

The Science of Safety and Connection

Humans are constantly seeking a state of safety and connection and, according to polyvagal theory (PVT), this originates not in the conscious, rational brain but in the primal, unconscious nervous system. PVT was described by Dr. Stephen Porges and brought into practical therapeutic situations by Deb Dana.[11] PVT is a way to befriend your biology.

The safety-seeking of the nervous system is governed by the vagus nerve, a cranial nerve exiting the base of the brain and meandering down, touching the heart, lungs, and digestive organs. Over time, the nervous system evolved, creating a hierarchy with the oldest iteration at the bottom and the newest at the top.

Five hundred million years ago, the nervous system protected you through immobilization, known in PVT as the *dorsal vagal complex*. When a life threat is detected, your biology goes into shutdown to conserve energy and hopefully outlast the threat. This state is associated with feeling dissociated, isolated, overwhelmed, ashamed, numb, helpless, and hopeless.

One hundred million years later, the nervous system evolved to mobilize against perceived threats. The *sympathetic nervous system* allowed you to fight or flee in the face of danger and has two channels: one associated with fear, including feelings of panic and anxiety, and one associated with anger, including frustration, irritation, and rage.

Most recently, although still 200 million years ago, the nervous system evolved to protect you through connection with others. Humans became pack animals, ensuring survival by being in relationship. The *ventral vagal complex* is where you feel most yourself: calm, curious, creative, confident, clear, courageous, compassionate, and connected.

These three states of the nervous system—with dorsal at the bottom, sympathetic in the middle, and ventral at the top—form the autonomic hierarchy. The nervous system is "regulated" when ventral is in charge and "dysregulated" when sympathetic or dorsal is running the show.

You can sense the states of your nervous systems based on the feelings and sensations you personally attribute to each state. Knowing the nervous system constantly and unconsciously scans for signs of safety and danger—known as neuroception—you can understand what your body is perceiving and how it is trying to protect you. With mindfulness, you can bring this unconscious perception into consciousness and cultivate more experiences of safety and connection.

A third aspect of PVT besides the hierarchy and neuroception is co-regulation. Co-regulation is when neuroception picks up signs of safety from other nervous systems—from other people. It anchors you into the regulated ventral vagal state. Co-regulation shows the importance of being in relationship to feel regulated.

MINDFUL MOMENT: Explore Your Own Autonomic Hierarchy

According to polyvagal theory, mindfulness can enhance your awareness of the different states you move through on any given day. This, in itself, can support Intuitive Eating. Here is an example of how I experience the three levels of my autonomic hierarchy.

Dorsal: Physically sleepy, body feels heavy and wooden, sensation of caving into myself. Emotionally shameful, feeling alienated from others, feeling "cursed," wanting to disappear.

Sympathetic: Physical muscle tension, jaw clenched, tightness in chest and throat, knot in stomach, buzzy sensation in lips and upper arms, might crave crunching on chips or corn nuts. Emotional overwhelm, feeling trapped, thinking speeds up, can't make sense of my thoughts, lost perspective, no distinction between irritants and catastrophes.

Ventral: Physically open sensation in chest, no tension in the jaw, abdomen relaxed, lips and arms feel neutral, body feels relaxed. Emotionally interested in my experience and in others' experience, content and satisfied, able to work with difficulty, open to feeling, flow, engaged with the world, feeling squarely in my own life, confidence that everything will be okay.

In your journal, explore your own autonomic hierarchy by contemplating how you feel when shut down (dorsal), activated into fight or flight (sympathetic), and peaceful and connected (ventral). For each state, what physical sensations and emotions do you experience?

As you move through your day, notice when you feel you are in different states. Ask yourself the questions from the Checking In with Yourself practice from chapter 1 to clarify what you are feeling and how you know. Consider setting a calendar reminder to do this exercise again in three months to see if your awareness has changed.

By becoming familiar with your states, physically and emotionally, you can do several things: recognize your body's responses to situations, understand triggers for fight-or-flight or shutdown responses, and discover ways to change dysregulated states into a state of safety and connection.

Connection, Belonging, and Diet Culture

Connection and belonging are important to feeling safe in your body and the world. So it makes sense you are deeply impacted by the images and messages of diet culture. While the overt incentive of diet culture is supposedly about health promotion (spoiler alert: it is not!), the covert objective is to sell products and services. The tagline is essentially, "Buy this and feel love, acceptance, and a sense of belonging!" When you are driven to feel connected and safe, and the predominant culture convinces you the only way is to be thin, then dieting becomes a form of survival.

MINDFUL MOMENT: How Diet Culture Affects Your Nervous System

In this exercise, you will expose yourself to images of diet culture. Notice the immediate impact of these images and messages on your nervous system, then give that impact a name. Please use your judgment as to whether this exercise is right to do today. Approach your nervous system with a sense of curiosity and respect. If it would be too triggering, skip this exercise and come back another day. Also, only do this exercise if you have time to complete the Intuitive Eating Glimmers exercise coming up, so you finish this chapter in a ventral state.

Grab your journal and plan to look at images promoting diet culture, such as thinspiration or fitspiration accounts on social media, the pages of a fashion or lifestyle magazine, or advertisements for a diet program, gym, or medical "beauty" spa. As you look at the images, ask:

- What sensations arise in your body?

- What emotions do you experience?

- Could you give them specific names?

- What actions do you notice you want to take? For example, you may go into shutdown and feel hopeless. Or you might want to spring into action and "get back on track."

- Does your experience feel like the dorsal state of shutdown or the sympathetic state of fight or flight? Or are you able to anchor into the ventral state and see the flawed logic in these images? Perhaps you experience all these states, to some extent.

Call to mind how your nervous system is always trying to protect you. Contemplate how even dysregulated reactions to images of diet culture are a form of that protection. Journal about what that is like.

Connection, Belonging, and Intuitive Eating

Intuitive Eating is an embodied process. It can be understood intellectually, but it only takes root when you feel it in your body. You must feel safe enough to engage your body. A nervous system preoccupied with fighting, fleeing, or freezing cannot reasonably be expected to deepen attunement and compassion.

Intuitive Eating, sharpened through mindfulness, anchors you in the ventral state, where you feel regulated and like yourself. Here, relationship is key. It begins with you. See if you can rouse senses of connection and belonging within your body. Place your hand on your heart and feel your own warmth, the warmth of the body you've lived in your whole life. The body that cares for you in infinite invisible ways. While it feels fraught to connect with your body, all relationships are hard. They are also immensely rewarding.

Now consider you and I are in relationship. I believe in your capacity for self-regulation, your ability to tolerate discomfort and learn from it, your discernment of what is happening in your body, mind, and heart. I see past the confusion diet culture has created, to your core goodness. And I know when you connect with that and are authentically yourself, the world benefits.

Finally, consider the millions who get caught in the diet culture's web, many of whom are now on their own Intuitive Eating path. You may never know them, but consider forming a relationship with them in your heart based on trust in your innately intelligent body.

When you are anchored in the ventral—safe and connected—state, you are said to be receiving "glimmers" of hope, connection, and warmth. Glimmers are a wonderful description of the sometimes-fleeting moments of peace and flow as you embark on an Intuitive Eating path. You may prefer to feel this sense of safety in large chunks. I would too. But the reality is they begin as little tastes. Recognizing those little tastes contributes to greater experiences in the future.

MINDFUL MOMENT: Intuitive Eating Glimmers

Get that journal again. Settle into your body and notice any sensations and emotions. Read the passage below, which is the authors' dedication at the beginning of the fourth edition of *Intuitive Eating*:

> We dedicate this book to our past and present clients and future Intuitive Eaters, and to the health professionals doing this work:
>
> May you have dignity, health, and happiness—regardless of your body size or shape.
>
> May you never doubt your inner wisdom or experience.

Reading these words, what glimmers arise? What feels hopeful and inspiring? What images come to mind? Words? Emotions? Sensations?

As you continue your Intuitive Eating practice, record your glimmers: a perfect bite of food, the certainty of knowing exactly what you are craving, the exhilaration of a pleasurable sensation, recognizing a difficult emotion without trying to escape it. Collect them like seashells and review them periodically.

Deepening Awareness

Stabilizing your nervous system sharpens real-time awareness of what is happening in your body.[12] Your body continuously communicates with you about hunger, fullness, comfort, pain, temperature, energy level, emotional state, and more. Paying mindful attention to those messages makes your Intuitive Eating practice sensitive, receptive, and precisely responsive.

Mindfulness brings unconscious perception (neuroception) into conscious awareness.[13] If, for example, your nervous system detects some threatening aspect of diet culture, mindfulness may help you notice your body reacting and understand any subsequent sensations, thoughts, emotions, or actions.

Sense What's Happening in Your Body

Interoception is this capacity to sense and interpret what is happening in your body in real time. It is a core concept in both Intuitive Eating and mindfulness.[3] Interoception is related to hunger, fullness, needing to pee, and feeling a headache coming on. But it extends far beyond the physical.

You were born with interoception. As a baby, interoception caused you to cry when you were uncomfortable in a wet diaper, to cry in a different way when you were hungry, and to turn away from the breast or bottle once you were full and satisfied. Interoception makes Intuitive Eating a true mind-body practice.

Initially, Intuitive Eating requires unlearning everything you thought you knew about food, health, and weight and relearning something entirely different. It can be mind-bending to imagine your body does not need to be monitored, manipulated, and controlled to discover well-being.

Consider this: most of us associate pink with girls and blue with boys. But did you know the reverse used to be the case? In the early 1900s, when sex-specific colors first emerged, pink was for boys, while the more delicate blue was for girls. Imagining that boy is not inherently blue and girl is not unilaterally pink might make your head spin. Like the idea you can self-regulate with Intuitive Eating, it may be hard for your conditioned mind to grasp at first.

Truly understanding Intuitive Eating might require you to consciously flip automatic thoughts around. When you feel the impact of feeding yourself according to hunger and fullness in your body, Intuitive Eating becomes more natural. You don't have to do the mental machinations to get there.

Mindfulness practices such as meditation, breath work, and yoga sharpen interoception. They reduce distractions, allowing a specific object to come into focus. In shamatha-vipashyana meditation, introduced in chapter 1, that object is the feeling of the breath. In your Intuitive Eating practice, the "object" is generally your present-moment body. Sometimes it is the sensations of hunger. Other times it is fullness or satisfaction. And much of the time it is the sensations of emotions in the body. Ultimately, interoception is how your body's unconscious perceptions become conscious. When you are conscious in your body, you can respond to needs with precision and kindness.

Shelby's Story

Shelby's mom always focused on her appearance. Shelby learned from a young age that her looks were the most important thing about her. So she looked to others to tell her how she was doing, whether she was making the right choices, and what and when and how much to eat. Unsurprisingly, she struggled to trust her own body and had a story about herself that she didn't know how to take care of herself. Tuning in to interoception, Shelby found evidence that she did, in fact, know how to take care of herself, for example, when she:

- *Was hungry after work but too tired to cook so she picked up takeout from her favorite Chinese restaurant.*

- *Recognized a moment of extreme stress at work that normally would have triggered emotional eating and instead did some mindful breathing.*

- *Adjusted meal times, frequency, and amounts in response to temporary gastrointestinal issues.*

- *Noticed a desire to connect with others to support herself through grief.*

Mindful attunement to interoception proved to Shelby that she was wise and capable of self-care.

MINDFUL MOMENT: Explore What You Sense in Your Body

Come to a comfortable lying-down position. Gently close your eyes or keep them slightly open. Moving at your own pace, begin at the bottom of your body and move up to the top:

Notice any sensations in the toes: temperature, pain, pleasure, neutral sensations.

Move up to the tops and bottoms of your feet, ankles, calves and shins, fronts and backs of your knees, tops of the thighs, backs of the thighs, buttocks, hips, pelvis, lower belly, lower back, middle belly, middle back, upper belly, chest, upper back, shoulders, upper arms, forearms, hands, fingers, neck, face, sides of the head, back of the head, top of the head.

Use your journal to record "noticings." Bring this mindful moment into the rest of your life by realizing when unconscious bodily experiences become conscious. Can you identify the moment you realize you need to pee? The moment you realize you are hungry, full, satisfied, tired, angry, happy, nervous, excited? How do you know? You may notice sensations arising as you read through this book. Your body is always communicating with you.

A classic phrase states "the mind is as the brain does." It describes how the structure and function of the brain influence how you experience your life. Changes in your brain brought about by mindfulness such as meditation engender feelings of presence, patience, and kindness, toward yourself and toward others. Your stabilized nervous system makes changing habitual patterns more accessible, and deepened interoception hones self-literacy.

What Can You Celebrate?

- What did you learn in this chapter?

- What did you confirm?

- Where do you have greater awareness of your physical body?

- Where do you have greater awareness of your emotions?

CHAPTER 3

Hunger

Hunger is a wonderful point to jump into or deepen an Intuitive Eating practice. Physical sensations of hunger help you connect with your body, sense and interpret nuance, accept uncertainty, and rebuild trust and confidence in yourself. Mindfulness sharpens attunement to hunger, and feeding your body as it wishes to be fed fuels the capacity for mindfulness.

The Importance of Eating Enough

The most important place to begin an Intuitive Eating practice is to ensure you are eating enough. Many people are surprised by the assertion they might not be eating enough because they are convinced their problem is eating too much. But insensitivity to physical cues of hunger, intentional or unintentional restriction, and inconsistent eating over the course of the day may mean your body is not getting enough nutrition.

To be clear, eating enough means you eat regularly throughout the day. You eat adequately at each meal and snack. You consume a balance of protein, carbohydrate, and fat, each of which meets the body's needs in a different way. And you allow yourself to eat the foods you like.

Because the body is hardwired to seek food until its needs are met, being chronically underfed will undercut efforts to reestablish trust and confidence in your body's self-regulation. It will also distort efforts to eventually work with the emotional side of your relationship with food. Only when you are adequately fed can you truly understand and embody Intuitive Eating.

This is a lot, I know, and we will break this down as we go. For now, try to absorb this fact: before getting into the deeper emotional aspects of your relationship with food and body, you must meet your basic biological needs. You must eat enough!

Also know eating enough can be complicated by the conflicting messages of diet culture, which has a lot to say about what, when, and how much you should eat. Those messages caused you to focus on how to manipulate timing of meals, to override natural signals of hunger and fullness, to question what you crave, and to prioritize "dietary correctness" (whatever the current iteration may be) over attunement to your body's ever-changing needs.

Narrowing your focus to sensations of hunger helps you fend off and unlearn confusing diet culture messages while stabilizing your body and preparing it for the subtler work of Intuitive Eating. Connecting with hunger is the entry point to true embodiment.

Hunger Across the Spectrum

Hunger is one of many ways your body communicates with you. When you notice sensations of hunger, you can tune in, interpret, and respond as best as you can. You become familiar with the full spectrum of your hunger, from not at all hungry to the hungriest you've ever felt, and make connections between the hunger level at which you begin to eat and the eating experience you have as a result. Ultimately, you can choose to eat at the hunger level at which you have the most enjoyable eating experience.

Recognizing hunger across the spectrum is the foundation for the other Intuitive Eating principles. It allows you to collect the data proving your body can be trusted.

The Physiology of Hunger

Understanding the physiology of hunger helps you connect the dots between sensations, decisions, and resultant eating experiences. Hunger sensations are directly related to your body's need for energy. Think of hunger as a continuum with "not hungry" at one end and "the hungriest

I've ever felt" at the other. When "not hungry," your body's need for energy is temporarily met. When you're "the hungriest I've ever felt," your body is communicating an extreme need for energy.

Where you are on the hunger spectrum is never perfectly static. Imagine a ball on a wire slowly moving from one end to the other and then back again. That ball is always moving as the body's need for energy emerges, as you eat, as the body utilizes that energy for bodily processes, and as the body remains sated for some time (with lots of bodily functions happening in the background), and then the process begins all over again.

The Sensations of Hunger

Different levels of hunger manifest as sensations. "Not hungry" may feel like an absence of sensation or a neutral feeling. "Gently hungry" may be an empty feeling. "Moderately hungry" may include grumbling or gurgling noises in the belly and thoughts of food. "Extremely hungry" could turn painful. All of this is your body's way of communicating with you.

How your body feels hunger is unique to you, though there are some commonalities. Hunger tends to show up in the following places:

- Mouth: preoccupation with the mouth, desire for oral stimulation, urge to put food in the mouth, mouth watering

- Throat/esophagus: achiness, dull pain, gnawing sensation

- Stomach: emptiness, hunger pangs, gurgling, gnawing, nausea, pain

- Head: difficulty concentrating, fogginess, sleepiness, light-headedness, headache, persistent thoughts of food

- Emotional: irritability, moodiness, flat affect, impatience, hungry + angry = hangry

Most of us associate hunger with the stomach, but many people rarely or never feel hunger there. Understanding how different levels of hunger show up for you is key to an attuned, responsive relationship with your body.

MINDFUL MOMENT: Hunger Meditation

Sit up straight wherever you are, balancing alertness with relaxation. Close your eyes gently or leave them open with a soft gaze. Bring awareness to the following areas:

- *Mouth:* What do you notice? Does it feel dry? Salivating? Do any sensations stand out? Are they positive, negative, or neutral? Does your mouth crave a sensory experience or does it feel satisfied for now?

- *Throat/esophagus:* What sensations are present? Do they change as you continue to pay attention? What is it like to relax this part of your body? Have you ever paid attention to it before?

- *Stomach:* What sensations are present? Are they positive, negative, or neutral? Let your awareness rest here for a few minutes and notice whether sensations emerge, surge, and then recede, or change in any way.

- *Head:* What sensations, perceptions, or preoccupations do you notice here?

- *Emotional:* What emotions are you aware of? Where are they? Do you feel tense, restless, peaceful, content, flat, heavy, light, speedy, impatient? Simply notice.

Record any "noticings" in your journal. This hunger meditation can be done before you eat or any time. When you regularly eat at a comfortable level of hunger, it is easier to remember to do this practice. It is a way to be with your body and become familiar with nuances of physical hunger. It is useful in the morning for people who are "never hungry for breakfast." You may wish to try it in times, locations, or situations that trigger eating in the absence of physical hunger, such as after a satisfying dinner.

The more aware of and responsive to hunger sensations, the more precisely you can meet your body's needs for energy. The less aware and responsive, the more confusing hunger feels and the more distorted your relationship with food and your body.

MINDFUL MOMENT: Create Your Personalized Hunger Scale

Organizing sensations of hunger in a personalized hunger scale helps you inter-pret them. When you notice emerging hunger and prioritize eating at that "sweet spot," you can have the most enjoyable and peaceful eating experience.

Write the numbers 1 to 10 in your journal. Choose whether they go horizon-tally or vertically. Number 1 represents the absence of hunger. Number 10 is the hungriest you've ever felt.

Beginning with number 10, what are the sensations of your most extreme hunger in your mouth, throat, esophagus, stomach, head, and emotions? What thoughts and emotions are present? How do those thoughts and emotions support or conflict with your ability to feed yourself according to your needs?

Go to the opposite end of the scale. What does not hungry feel like in your body? This is different from fullness, which exists on a separate scale and is covered in the next chapter. How do you know whether you are not hungry? Is the absence of sensation a sensation itself? Perhaps you notice a neutral sensa-tion, as if there is nothing in particular happening.

For each remaining point on the scale, capture the sensory experience you feel. This exercise is less about deciphering between a 2.5 or a 3 and more about recognizing hunger moving across a spectrum.

How Hunger Level Affects Your Eating Experience

Another brief physiology lesson. Your body is hardwired to seek food when in need of energy, so food tastes best when you are moderately hungry. I think of this as numbers 4 through 6 on a 1-to-10 hunger scale, but it may be slightly higher or lower for you. When moderately hungry, you are most likely to detect what you are craving, to eat at an enjoyable pace, to enjoy your food, to notice emerging fullness and subtle taste changes as you eat, and to stop at a point you deem "enough."

Below the moderately hungry range, when your appetite is less physi-cally driven, eating may still be pleasurable but it may not follow the typical arc described above. Intuitive Eating gives you unconditional permission to eat, including in the absence of physical hunger. When you do choose to eat at this point in the hunger scale, pay attention. Notice your expectations and your actual experience. Be honest, gentle, and compassionate. And when you experiment with "charged" foods that provoke strong emotional reactions, you may wish to be lower on the hunger scale, for example, at a level between 1 and 3.

When extremely hungry, in the 7 to 10 range of the hunger scale, eating feels different than when moderately or not at all hungry. At this extreme level, you may crave foods differently and/or have trouble identifying what you are hungry for. For example, if you wanted a burger when you were moderately hungry but didn't stop to eat, by the time you reach extreme hunger, you might crave something more easily broken down into sugar for the body, like candy.

When you eat at this "primal" level of hunger, your body's priority is to get the food in. You are likely to eat more quickly and to miss out on the sensory experience of what you're eating, which may cost you enjoyment. You might miss the subtle cues of emerging fullness, and you may eat past the point of "comfortable fullness."

If you didn't understand this is a normal response to extreme hunger, eating when exceptionally hungry may become a binge. If possible, avoid this danger zone of extreme hunger, especially when you are new to Intuitive Eating.

Sometimes it is impossible to avoid extreme hunger, so please be gentle with yourself. If you find yourself here, know it is normal to be drawn to carbohydrates, to eat quickly, and to overeat. Pay attention to your eating experience in these moments, but don't be hard on yourself if you simply cannot stay present. If you binge, don't panic. Do not restrict to compensate for a binge. Acknowledge it happened and remind yourself you still need to eat.

Gaia's Story

Gaia was a busy pediatrician with two children under three and a husband who traveled for work, frequently leaving her alone with the kids. Gaia was a chronic dieter who was often trapped in the cycle of restrict-binge-restrict. We soon discovered Gaia was consistently undereating during the day, which set her up for binges later in the afternoon and evening when family demands were greatest and patience and resilience were wearing thin. To offset this, she increased her intake earlier in the day and ensured she was getting a balance of protein, carbohydrate, and fat. For the most part, Gaia's bingeing dissipated.

During a particularly brutal week at work and home, Gaia binged even though she was eating adequately. Between appointments, she emailed that as uncomfortable as she was with bingeing, she knew giving in to restriction would reignite the cycle. Instead, Gaia used mindfulness, acceptance, and self-compassion to acknowledge what happened, offer herself kindness, and remind herself she still needed to eat regularly the next day. This was the first time she binged without getting sucked back into that cycle.

MINDFUL MOMENT: Experiment with Hunger

Once you have a feel for your own hunger spectrum, notice the eating experiences you have when beginning at different levels. Depending on where you are in your hunger scale, how easily can you recognize what you're craving? How fast do you eat? How satisfied are you with your choices? How present are you? Do you notice any taste changes as you eat? Do you notice emerging fullness? Are you able to recognize the point of "enough"?

What is your "sweet spot" of hunger? At what level of hunger do you have the most enjoyable eating experience? Usually, this is somewhere in the middle of the scale, at which you are hungry enough for food to taste good but not so hungry that eating becomes chaotic and mindless.

Come back to this exercise over time. You might find the results change each time you do it. You might even wish to revise your hunger scale. Early in this process, for example, some people think 5 is their sweet spot. As they continue to notice their eating experiences, however, they may prefer to begin at a gentler level of hunger.

If you do this experiment when not at all hungry or in the danger zone of hunger, try to use the experience to notice and collect data. Ask yourself the same questions above. Could you view the experience not as right or wrong, but as an opportunity to learn?

Hunger Distortions

Many things can disrupt natural hunger cues. Sickness, stress, lack of sleep, time zone changes—all can confuse the body and change how and when hunger sensations emerge. Chronic busyness, a history of restriction, frequently skipping meals, anxiety or depression, and certain medications can also prevent you from recognizing hunger and eating regularly. This is another example of how the body and the mind are connected: when your body is stressed for any reason, it changes how you experience your life, including how you feel hunger.

Other things that can distort hunger include the use of caffeine or nicotine, both of which are appetite suppressants. Many people who claim to not experience hunger in the morning may in fact be masking those sensations by drinking a cup (or three) of coffee. I would never suggest you stop drinking coffee (perish the thought!), but if you do enjoy a cup, eat some breakfast with it or directly afterward and see how that affects the rest of your day regarding energy, mood, cravings, and the quality and quantity of your eating experiences.

If you have tended toward restrained eating earlier in the day that leads to eating larger quantities in the evening, you may not feel hunger in the morning. How to work with this is to shift your eating to be more balanced over the course of the day. This may involve eating breakfast a few times in the absence of hunger, but with attention, practice, and patience, your intake will ultimately equilibrate.

Interim Option: Structured Approaches to Eating

If you initially feel overwhelmed at the blank slate of an Intuitive Eating practice, "structured eating" may help. A structure may also be useful if you are not yet experiencing clear hunger signals, if you tend to skip meals and snacks, or if your schedule prevents you from naturally eating regularly.

Structured eating entails eating approximately every three to four hours, with a combination of protein, carbohydrate, and fat, even if you're not particularly hungry. Organizing your meals and snacks like this provides a scaffolding that supports you to become more attuned to your actual needs. It allows your body to have the experience of eating regularly and adequately and prevents your hunger from veering toward the danger zone, which can lead to binge eating. This might elicit dormant hunger signals so you can become more familiar with their nuances.

A typical structure is breakfast, lunch, snack, and dinner. But there is no need to be typical when it comes to eating. Your only obligation is to yourself. What works for your life? Your schedule? Your family and their schedule?

For example, if you like to exercise first thing in the morning but find yourself excessively hungry afterward, perhaps a snack before your workout, breakfast after your workout, then lunch, afternoon snack, and dinner is the right pattern for you. If you prefer to eat smaller more frequent meals throughout the day and dinner with your family, maybe snack, snack, snack, snack, dinner is your pattern.

Experiment with different eating patterns and design different options for different days. You might have one structure when you work from home and another when you commute. You might have one structure on the days you go for hikes with a friend and another on the days you do yoga at home.

When you practice structured eating, always default to your body's needs to define what you eat, when, and how much. Choose foods that appeal to you in the moment rather than those supposed to be health-promoting. If hunger signals precede the timing of the next structured meal or snack, take note and default to your body's requests. The structure is there to support and protect you, but your body's clear signals should take precedence. This is how you transition from a structure to your own genuine Intuitive Eating.

Return to structured eating whenever you experience disruptions that make it hard to meet your body's needs in real time. Whether on vacation, sick, or during a particularly stressful period, eating regularly and consistently according to a structure will support your physiologic stability, mental resilience, and cognitive flexibility. Pay attention with open, gentle curiosity and be willing to break from your plan when your body communicates it needs something different.

The Need for Compromise

When beginning an Intuitive Eating journey, ideally you would eat exactly what you want at your precise sweet spot of hunger. In reality, however, you probably have to balance Intuitive Eating with a work schedule, family meals, subpar options when your first choice is unavailable, and various real-life inconveniences. All of this is totally workable.

The point of Intuitive Eating isn't perfection. It's awareness and flexibility. Great if you can eat exactly what you want when you want it. Also great if you aren't able to because that gives you more information. Try to see working with hunger as an ongoing conversation and a series of compromises in which you work together with your body and in your real life. Eventually you will navigate the subtleties of hunger so you are close to where you want to be for various eating experiences.

MINDFUL MOMENT: Checking In with Hunger

To continually sharpen your sensitivity to hunger, come back to the following questions. Use your journal to record "noticings" and check back in with previous answers:

- How often do I notice hunger emerging?

- How frequently am I in the danger zone before noticing hunger?

- What is happening for me/around me when I get into the danger zone?

- How often do I respond to my hunger when I notice it?

- How often do I know what I'm hungry for?

- What does my "sweet spot" of hunger feel like?

- How do I know?

MINDFUL MOMENT: Flashing Mindfulness

When you don't have time for a formal meditation practice, a planned hunger check-in, or the full hunger meditation, you can always "flash" mindfulness. Whenever you are suddenly aware of yourself in the present moment—with mind and body in the same place at the same time—acknowledge this synchronicity. Hold your body with restful dignity. Release expectations of yourself and your experience. Bring your awareness to your sensual body—sensations, sights, sounds, smells, tastes, textures—and for just a few moments *be*.

Messy Mindful Eating

Many people think mindful eating is about being perfectly placid and meditative every moment of an eating experience, in a way that excludes relaxation, emotions, and thoughts. If this were the case, I would *never* practice mindful eating. Boring!

I encourage people to practice messy and imperfect mindful eating, which, by the way, is the only true mindful eating. Imperfect mindful eating leaves room for being human, with little bits of effort and awareness that culminate in greater presence and appreciation of eating.

Messy mindful eating includes:

- Minimizing distractions, even if this means turning off devices for just the first five minutes or first five bites of an eating experience

- Taking small steps to enhance enjoyment of an eating experience, for example, by using a favorite bowl or altering the lights in a way that feels good for your nervous system

- Taking a moment to acknowledge the good fortune of having a human body, of having food to eat, of enjoying the fruits of the labor of countless individuals you will never meet (farmers, drivers, factory workers, supermarket personnel, etc.)

- Directing attention to the sensual body, noticing how the body feels generally, as well as focusing on the senses of taste, smell, appearance, sound, and texture

- Savoring the food and the experience, which begins with simply noticing

Practicing any of the points above—even if not all of them at the same time—*counts* as mindful eating. Messy mindful eating can happen anywhere and at any point in an eating experience. If you eat a meal and only with the last bite notice you haven't been paying attention, take that one bite with awareness—and without judgment. I personally have mindfully enjoyed many a spoonful of Nutella standing over the kitchen sink. The point is not to strive for perfection but to simply show up in your own life.

Your exploration of your body's communication begins with hunger, but eventually you can sense more subtle physical states, including those associated with emotions. This is how working with hunger ultimately transforms your entire relationship with your body. Hunger protects you and anchors you in your body. Mindfulness keeps you in touch with that and supports you every step of the way.

What Can You Celebrate?

- What did you notice about your own experience with hunger?

- What connections did you make regarding your hunger scale and the types of eating experiences you have?

- What have you decided to pay attention to?

CHAPTER 4

Fullness

When you are eating enough, stopping at the point of comfortable fullness becomes a form of self-care (and, dare I say, pleasure!). Just as never letting yourself experience fullness is not working with the reality of your body's needs, neither is chronically overshooting it. In this chapter, you will learn how to respect fullness with precision and gentleness.

Working with fullness can be challenging, so please be kind and patient with yourself. Your exploration of fullness might need to come a little later in the process. It may not work for you to address fullness directly after you address hunger, as the order of these chapters would suggest. It may be best to read through the other aspects of your Intuitive Eating practice before coming back to fullness. Listen to your wise body, mind, and heart to guide you.

Fullness Is a Form of Communication, and Mindfulness Helps You Hear

Fullness is another way the body communicates. It is part of the call and response between body and mind: the body feels sensations and the mind interprets them, enabling you to respond. Mindfulness practices help with this interpretation, allowing you to notice when something has changed, understand in real time what is needed, and take action. Mindfulness also helps you evaluate—without judgment—whether a particular choice worked well or not so you can make a different choice given a similar situation in the future.

Because mindfulness is paying attention in a certain way, mindfulness of fullness requires patient attunement to notice real-time changes in the body as you eat. The attention you pay to fullness must be infused with gentleness. This gentleness will accompany you throughout your life and assist you whenever you encounter emotionally fraught obstacles.

Why Fullness Is Challenging

Hunger sensations often feel concrete. Emptiness, hunger "pangs," gurgling, and even the nausea of extreme hunger communicate the body's need to eat. Plus, it feels good to have permission to eat. Heeding your body's signals of hunger feels like a relief.

Working with fullness, on the other hand, relates to stopping eating. When you were dieting, stopping eating was always the focus. It's no wonder, then, that working with fullness in Intuitive Eating can initially feel fraught. This demonstrates how the way you *feel* about an aspect of the process affects the process. And it's a reminder that Intuitive Eating is a nonlinear process that should be done at your own pace.

Before discovering Intuitive Eating, you probably rarely asked yourself what "comfortable fullness" felt like. Because the diet culture taught you not to trust your body to tell you when it had enough, you thought internal cues would lead you astray and instead relied on external criteria to tell you how much to eat. This might have led you to a fullness level that was wrong for you—too little due to extreme caution or too much to rebel against limitations.

By prioritizing external over internal factors like how the food tastes and how your body feels, fullness remained a mysterious target you never hit. This is not surprising. When the message is to eat as little as possible, how can you ever feel you are getting the right amount?

Internal Cues of Fullness

In the next chapter, you will learn about satisfaction and how it is different from and complementary to fullness. Here, think of fullness as occurring in different body parts: the mouth, stomach, and general body and mind. It is the constellation of what you experience in these body parts that helps you understand emerging fullness.

Mouth

One of the first signs your body is becoming full is a subtle change in the taste of food. Because your body is wired to find food the most appealing when moderately hungry—somewhere in the middle of your hunger scale—as hunger dwindles, so too do the pleasure signals in the brain. Another sensation occurring in the mouth is less urge to put food in. This happens for the same reason as diminishing pleasure signals of taste.

Even though signs of fullness occurring in the mouth are some of the earliest, allow yourself to realize this in your own time. This is something you cannot rush. Trust that you will experience it when your awareness and sense of security are ready.

At times, you might fight the awareness of mouth fullness and wish to continue the pleasant experience of eating. It is fine if you notice the change in taste or the desire to eat but wish to override it. What's important is that you notice. Eventually, you'll be ready to experiment with stopping according to internal signals.

Stomach

The most common sign of fullness occurs in the stomach. Stretch or distention is caused by the quantity of food in the stomach. As you eat, the degree of stretch increases.

Stretch in the stomach is more about the volume of food than the energy density of the food or how nourishing it is. Carbohydrate, protein, and fat provide the greatest energy (caloric) density. Foods high in fiber and water may feel more filling but don't provide as much energy as something denser but with less volume.

When you don't manipulate food for weight loss or maintenance and you eat a variety of foods, the sensation of stretch can be one useful data point in deciding when to stop eating. However, fullness *is* commonly manipulated for the purposes of dieting.

One diet capitalized on the filling capacity of foods with very few calories. *Volumetrics* was a type of "eat this, not that" diet that helped you feel full on fewer calories. A Volumetrics-friendly choice would be a bowl of soup containing broth, vegetables, and chicken. Because it contains a lot of water and fiber but not much carbohydrate and fat, you are likely to feel stretch in the stomach without many calories.

On the other hand, if you eat something with greater energy density and less water and fiber, like an energy bar, it will take up less space in your stomach. This would cause less stretch even though the food may be more nourishing. In this example, the fullness from the soup wouldn't last and you would likely get hungry sooner. Even though the energy bar didn't "fill you up," you might feel sated for some time because of the energy density.

General Body and Mind

Certain sensations happen in the general body and mind as fullness emerges. These changes are different from thoughts and feelings, though they often overlap. Sensations occurring in the general body and mind are the direct result of the body's physiologic need for energy being met.

Many people notice a "relaxation response" that arises as they reach fullness. If hunger (particularly if chronically unattended to) is a sign of danger, then fullness can be regarded as a sign of safety. As fullness emerges, you might notice physical release and relief—unclenching the muscles, relaxing the jaw, leaning back from the table, and feeling spacious (as opposed to tense) so you can suddenly think of things other than food.

Because hunger can involve preoccupation with food, with fullness your thoughts can go elsewhere. In the next two sections of this book, you will learn more about mindfulness of feelings and mindfulness of mind (or thoughts). For now, know that when you work toward unconditional permission to eat and consciously and regularly counter diet thoughts, your awareness of changes that happen with fullness will be clearer.

MINDFUL MOMENT: Create Your Own Fullness Scale

Just as you did with hunger, write the numbers 1 to 10 in your journal. Choose whether the numbers go horizontally or vertically. Number 1 represents the absence of fullness in your body. Number 10 is the fullest you've ever felt.

Beginning with number 10, what sensations did you feel when you were the fullest you can remember? Run through the parts of the body where fullness can be felt—mouth, stomach, general body—and note what you felt at this extreme level of fullness.

Now go to the opposite end of the scale. What does not at all full feel like in your body? Remember this is different from hunger, which exists on a separate scale. Do you notice an absence of sensation, a neutral sensation, or something else?

For each of the remaining points on the scale, describe what you feel. Just like hunger, this exercise is less about knowing the difference between a 7 and an 8 of fullness and more about recognizing how fullness emerges gradually and can be viewed as a spectrum. Within this spectrum, begin to contemplate what feels like your sweet spot of fullness. Notice whether you have different sweet spots for different circumstances.

MINDFUL MOMENT: Sitting with Fullness

In this short exercise, you'll simply sit with fullness—whatever level of fullness you happen to be at the moment. The next time you eat, assume a relaxed but upright posture and gently focus your awareness on the different parts of the body associated with fullness—mouth, stomach, general body and mind. In your journal, record your "noticings." What thoughts are present? How do you feel about being at this level of fullness? How do you feel about stopping at this point in the meal? As you experiment with different levels and different scenarios, return to this mindful moment to practice noticing.

Fullness Distortions

External criteria can override your understanding of fullness. One external criterion is the serving size printed on a package, like one ounce of potato chips; a "commonsense" serving size, like one-quarter of an avocado; or a unit of food, like one banana, one slice of pizza, or one piece of toast. Time limits on when you should eat, types of foods to be eaten at certain times or meals, and whether a food is allowed or off-limits in the first place can complicate fullness. These factors interfere with your ability to sense inward to determine whether and when you have reached that sweet spot.

Serving sizes don't care about you. This is because they have nothing to do with the individual doing the eating. They are arbitrary measures chosen because they are round numbers or based on some arcane production parameter. The idea that one ounce of potato chips is "the right amount" is useless. It doesn't reflect the different needs of different individuals or the needs of the same individual at different times. The same could be said about commonsense serving sizes, single-unit servings, appropriateness of the timing of eating or the types of foods eaten at different meals, and any form of red light, green light food rule.

Yet we love our 100-calorie packs and the idea of eating 1,200 calories per day. If you have this tendency to think in round numbers, consider it a manifestation of your wish for clarity, simplicity, and certainty. But also remember your needs are moving targets that change all the time.

MINDFUL MOMENT: Notice Your Fullness Cue Distorters

Grab your journal and read through this list of external cues that can distract from your internal ones. Identify which are prominent in your own eating experience:

- Serving sizes
- "Commonsense" servings
- Units of food
- How much of a food is available

- How much is served to you

- The size of the plate

- How much others are eating

- Time of day

- Others? Add your own!

As you work with fullness, notice when distortions interfere and consciously respond to them. When you notice how much others are eating, for example, acknowledge that, then redirect your attention to your internal cues to determine to what degree of fullness you wish to eat in that instance. Fullness distortions are not problems; they are reminders to mindfully engage with this confusion and to recommit your allegiance to your own intelligent body. Record your "noticings" in your journal and come back to them periodically.

When to Focus on Fullness

Before focusing on fullness, you must have total and unconditional permission to eat, you respond to your physical hunger more often than not, and you eat primarily for physical reasons (and have ways to cope with emotional hungers—see chapter 8). When you do these things with some consistency over time, you might become curious about eating to a more precise level of fullness.

Sometimes people notice when they have reached a certain point of fullness but continue to eat beyond that point. This is completely normal. Because dieting threatens the security of getting enough food, stopping when comfortably full can feel like deprivation. This is an interesting and complex point in the process that will unfold as you continue to pay attention.

If you are here, it is worth celebrating. You have noticed a part of your experience you didn't before. Paying attention to yourself in this nonjudgmental way is a form of true self-care. You have recognized fullness and chosen to continue eating, which is very different from eating beyond comfortable fullness without noticing. You have become curious about stopping at that point of fullness. And you are respecting your sense of readiness. Brava!

You may choose to stay here for some time. If you do, continue to notice as hunger diminishes, fullness emerges, and the constellation of sensations you feel point to that elusive sweet spot. If and when you notice dieting thoughts entering—*you should already be full, you should have stopped several bites ago*—respond with compassion. For example, "I am working on listening to my own body and its sensations, which are always changing. There is no *should* in fullness."

Giving yourself this degree of permission—full and unconditional permission—allows the emotional charge around fullness to dissipate and its distinction from deprivation to become clear. Eating to comfortable fullness confirms your capacity for Intuitive Eating, simply by paying attention with gentleness. Eventually, choosing to stop eating at "comfortable fullness" feels as accessible as continuing to eat.

You might feel compelled to explore the unfamiliar territory of stopping at a point you determine. Drop into your body to notice what is happening. Ask yourself, *How do I know I am at a point where I would like to stop? What data point me to this conclusion? How does it feel to imagine stopping now?* You don't have to feel 100 percent ready to try this, just "ready enough" to experiment.

When you feel ready, take a moment to remember that you always have permission to continue eating. Say to yourself, *I always have permission to eat. I am choosing to stop at this point to see how it feels and to learn what fullness means for my body in this moment.* What you do next is up to you. Two options are to get involved in some other activity, for example, taking a walk or reading a book, or to do some focused exploration of your experience, such as writing in your journal. You might try both options at different times.

After a few minutes, notice how you feel in your body. Where are you on the hunger scale? Where are you on the fullness scale? Are any emotions present, such as excitement, awe, anxiety, uncertainty, or restlessness? What does stopping at this point feel like in terms of self-care? How does stopping at this point impact your sense of pleasure?

Acknowledge the reality of your experience: what felt good, what felt challenging, and everything in between. What would you do the same? What would you do differently? You have the rest of your life to experiment with this, so give yourself the time and space to do so.

Once you have had the experience of stopping when comfortably full, that does not mean you can make only that choice going forward. Sometimes you will continue eating beyond comfortable fullness because the food tastes so good or simply because you want to. Sometimes you will pause and assess. And sometimes the choice to stop will feel crystal clear. All responses are good. There is no superiority to choosing to stop eating. The more you can emphasize this to yourself, the better. These are simply choices you make and opportunities to observe yourself.

Harley's Story

Harley never thought about her weight until she turned forty and went through surgical menopause. She gained weight around her belly, which made her ashamed. Harley began to restrict foods she thought caused weight gain but then felt out of control around those very foods. We discussed the need to address her physical and emotional needs with food. Physically, her body needed enough calories and a balance of protein, carbohydrate, and fat. Emotionally, she needed to give herself permission to eat the foods she craved or she would always be shadowboxing with herself. Over the next weeks Harley sent me several emails about her mindful experiments with unconditional permission and eating enough:

- *"Feeling and honoring my hunger, feeling less guilt about what I'm eating, continuing to read the research on dieting—very interesting!"*

- *"Ate pasta with Bolognese sauce and tossed salad—I ate half of my portion and felt quite full, so I waited to see if I wanted to eat more and I didn't. THIS IS THE FIRST TIME IN A LONG*

TIME I HAVE DONE THIS! *I usually keep eating just because it tastes good, or because I come to the table feeling starving."*

- *"Drank a box of organic apple juice at 10:30 a.m. NO GUILT. Tasted so good!!!!"*

- *"Paying attention and eating when hungry and stopping when full!!!!!!"*

- *"Undoing dieting rules I was trying to follow and then bingeing later...surprised at how much this was impacting my thoughts and feelings."*

MINDFUL MOMENT: Experiment with Fullness

This practice facilitates a deeper understanding of fullness in different situations. Start a section in your journal for these fullness experiments:

- Fullness in relation to hunger at the beginning of an eating experience:
  - When not very hungry, what degree of fullness do you prefer?
  - When moderately hungry, what degree of fullness do you prefer?
  - When primally hungry, to what degree of fullness do you tend to eat?

- Fullness in relation to meal composition:
  - To what degree of fullness do you choose to eat when your meal is "energy dense" (relatively low in water content and higher in fat and protein)?
  - To what degree of fullness do you choose to eat when your meal is primarily composed of carbohydrate?
  - To what degree of fullness do you choose to eat when your meal is higher in fat?
  - To what degree of fullness do you choose to eat when your meal is high in water content and fiber?

- Fullness in relation to drinking:

- How is fullness affected by drinking?
- Do you prefer to drink before, during, or after your meal?
- How is fullness affected by drinking alcohol?

- Fullness in relation to type of eating experience:
  - To what degree of fullness do you choose to eat when you are grazing throughout the day?
  - When you are celebrating a holiday or birthday?
  - When you are out at a restaurant?
  - When you are at a stand-up cocktail hour or buffet?

- Fullness in relation to other activities/seasons:
  - To what degree of fullness do you choose to eat before you exercise?
  - After you exercise?
  - In the colder months?
  - In the warmer months?
  - When you are not feeling well?

Your relationship with fullness may change over time. Sometimes you might stop at no longer hungry, other times you might habitually overshoot comfortable fullness. The most important part of this relationship is to continue to pay attention. And always speak to yourself with compassion.

What Can You Celebrate?

- What did you learn about fullness in this chapter?
- What did you notice about your own relationship with fullness?
- Is it time to work on this or are you not quite there yet? How do you know?
- What might signify readiness? What do you think you'll feel like when you're ready?

CHAPTER 5

Satisfaction, the Center of the Framework

In the third edition of *Intuitive Eating,* the authors placed satisfaction at the center of the other nine principles. Evelyn Tribole and Elyse Resch concluded this separately when they realized that having *enough*—feeling contented and tended to—liberates you to eat what you want, to the point that suits you in that moment. Once satisfied, you can move on with your life.

You may have become completely disconnected from the feeling of satisfaction, which is the feeling "I've had enough. My emotional and physical needs have been met. I feel content in this moment." With satisfaction at the center of the Intuitive Eating framework, what and how much you eat occupy their rightful place among your various and ever-changing preferences.

What Is Satisfaction?

Satisfaction cannot be predefined. You can understand what tastes, textures, temperatures, settings, and other factors contribute to satisfaction. But satisfaction is an in-the-moment experience. This is why mindfulness is key.

What satisfies you is separate from serving sizes or how much someone else needs to feel satisfied. Satisfaction is something only you can know. No one else can tell you when you are satisfied. And inherent in discovering satisfaction is the capacity to trust yourself—your body, your judgment.

Knowing you are satisfied feels different from knowing two plus two equals four. The *knowing* is somatic, not mathematical. Your body tells you when it's satisfied, but you must listen and feel. Perhaps your mouth no longer longs for subsequent bites. Your stomach feels content. Your heart-mind feels gratified, secure, and cared for. You feel no urgency for more.

You might initially think satisfaction comes from eating formerly forbidden foods. Or that it comes from eating as much as possible. Your understanding of satisfaction will unfold over time. Please allow this to happen and you will see that what truly satisfies you transcends the type or even amount of food you eat.

Satisfaction is a moving target and impossible to pin down with 100 percent certainty. When you feel satisfaction in your body, you can find balance with your eating, with movement, with your thoughts and feelings, and ultimately even with incorporating nutrition into your Intuitive Eating path.

In this chapter, we cover a lot of ground. First you will learn about the subtle but important differences between fullness and satisfaction. You'll discover the impacts of restrained versus permissive eating and what happens physically and emotionally with repeated exposures to the same tastes and textures. Finally, you will learn how to work with countless subtleties in centering satisfaction.

Fullness vs. Satisfaction

Fullness is primarily a physical experience representing the changes in the body as you continue to eat. The rewarding taste of food diminishes and the belly becomes full and somewhat stretched. The physical need for calories is met, so the body is not biologically driven to seek out more food.

You can attain fullness by eating a quantity of food, even if it's not food you like or want. But this type of eating experience would likely not produce a level of satisfaction. That comes from eating food you find delicious and, well, satisfying.

Satisfaction is more holistic than fullness. Fullness may be a component of satisfaction, for example, when you have chosen to eat what you want and you reach your sweet spot of comfortable fullness. Other times fullness and satisfaction may remain completely separate, as in the case of tasting someone's gelato but not craving one of your own.

When you are full but not satisfied, you might feel a bewildering desire for "something else." It is confusing to simultaneously feel a full belly and a longing for more. This scenario may initially represent a backlog of lost satisfaction. With practice, this will signify an eating experience did not meet your emotional needs even if it did meet your physical needs.

Kelsey's Story

Kelsey was a teacher who ate the school breakfasts and lunches. Her problem was after school. When she arrived home each day, Kelsey was exhausted and overwhelmed at the thought of cooking for herself. Diet mentality made food shopping painful, so she often ordered takeout, which not only consumed her paycheck but often didn't meet her expectations. Kelsey found herself compensating for the lack of quality by eating a greater quantity of that food.

Initially, Kelsey identified the foods she wanted to eat and sustainable ways to shop for, stock, and prepare them. Conveniences like grocery delivery, stocking plenty of easy, grab-and-eat options, and changing standards and expectations for "cooking" helped Kelsey feed herself consistently, satisfyingly, and with variety. She realized her evening meal coincided with needing "me time." The satisfaction she was seeking, therefore, was greater than what any food could reasonably provide. Kelsey reframed her satisfaction expectations for dinner and tended to her emotional needs with other self-care behaviors.

Satisfaction is related to three key concepts: restraint theory, habituation, and sensory-specific satiety. Understanding these concepts through a mindfulness lens will help you find satisfaction regularly.

Restraint Theory

Restraint theory was proposed in 1975 by researchers Hermann and Mack.[14] They found trying *not* to eat certain foods or certain quantities of food actually led to overeating. Restraint theory was based on observations that "restrained eaters" ate more (sometimes much more) than intended and many gained significant amounts of weight as a result. The "discipline, self-control, and willpower" exercised by many dieters, therefore, gave way to the opposite reaction. Perhaps you have experienced this for yourself?

Even when eating enough energy and macronutrients to meet your body's needs, restrained eating causes a backlash that derails attempts to control your food. When you feel deprived, ultimately you give in to perceived temptation. This leads to guilt and shame and more overeating. Eventually, you feel the need to reestablish control and reinstate those arbitrary limitations. It's not hard to see how this cycle could consume a significant portion of your life.

The antidote is to give yourself unconditional permission to eat. This may be a hard sell: even for those of us practicing in this field it can be difficult to accept that full and unconditional permission to eat is the secret to making peace with food. It shows you how deep and troubling programming by the diet culture has been, even for nutrition "experts." Unconditional permission to eat seems to contradict everything we were taught as dietitians and certainly as dieters. But there is radical wisdom in allowing yourself to eat what you want.

With unconditional permission to eat, there is no superior or inferior foods: all foods consist of different combinations of protein, carbohydrate, and fat with various sensory characteristics. Because there are no limitations, there's nothing to fight against. You can ask yourself, *What am I hungry for? What tastes, textures, and other sensory characteristics would satisfy me in this moment?*

Mindfulness both strengthens your self-literacy to help you choose what is satisfying and grounds you to tolerate new and uncertain experiences. This intuition is based on a constellation of factors that often defies explanation. And mindfulness helps you recognize when you are battling with your body and mind and supports you to thoughtfully change course.

Andrea's Story

Andrea never kept Oreos in the house. Any time they crossed the threshold, she binged on them. Once Andrea was eating regularly and had an adequate variety of foods stocked in the house, we addressed the Oreo situation. She agreed to always keep two or three boxes in the house. When one box was finished, she would buy another so there was never a threat of scarcity. If Andrea wanted Oreos when she wasn't physically hungry, she ate them with permission and attention—not distracting herself from the sensory experience and redirecting her attention to eating any time her attention strayed to thoughts like "I shouldn't be eating these." When Andrea was physically hungry and wanted Oreos, she agreed to eat them with the same attention and to complement them with some form of protein such as Greek yogurt. Understanding the physiology of satisfaction and giving herself consistent, unconditional permission to eat allowed Andrea to regard Oreos as just another food she enjoyed sometimes but that did not wield any special power over her.

MINDFUL MOMENT: What Is Your Own Experience with Restraint?

Grab your journal. What happened when you tried "restrained eating"? Do particular situations stand out for you? Whether you were trying to decrease the quantity of foods or avoiding particular foods, what did you notice about your physical experience of hunger? What did you choose to eat? How much did you eat? How satisfied did you feel? Did you want "something else"? Did you ever feel as though you had had enough? Did you eat what you originally craved in the end? What emotions were present? Draw your restrained eating cycle: connect the dots between restraint and what followed. What's it like to view your experience this way?

Habituation

If restraint is fueled by the fear you won't stop eating, then habituation is what happens when you do not arbitrarily limit yourself. It is a diminishing physical or emotional response to a frequently consumed food. Habituation happens naturally when you work toward unconditional permission to eat. When you are permitted to eat all foods regularly, eventually the charge around them drops. You can mindfully assist this process by becoming attuned to your needs and desires for specific quantities and qualities of foods. This attunement is built on the foundation of knowing you will have enough.

You might fear giving yourself unconditional permission to eat. The industries of diet culture make billions of dollars off you not trusting your body. Keep this in mind and be gentle, patient, and compassionate with yourself as you unlearn this lie.

Allowing habituation to unfold is a leap of faith. It is a direct challenge to everything you've been taught about food, eating, and your body based on a hope and belief in a different way. Any time you doubt your ability for habituation, return your attention to the process—to your body in the present moment or the eating experience happening right now—to gather supportive evidence from your own life. You were born with self-regulation; this is all about reconnecting with that innate wisdom.

Habituation happens with all foods, but can be particularly evident with emotionally "charged" foods, such as those forbidden fruits you so vehemently denied yourself. Continuing to expose yourself to these foods—giving yourself permission to eat them and paying attention to the sensory characteristics of the food—helps them assume their rightful place on the same moral plane as every other food.

In the early days of eating previously forbidden foods, the pendulum may swing from the extreme of restraint to the opposite extreme of unchecked eating. This is completely normal. An unrealistic expectation is that the pendulum can come to an abrupt halt right in the middle of its range as opposed to swinging back and forth a few times before gradually finding middle ground.

If, when you first experiment with charged foods, eating feels out of control, please resist the temptation to restrict or blame food addiction. The studies on food addiction do not stand up to critical analysis and they don't reflect the paradoxical relationship between restraint and overeating. Restrained eating will always increase your desire for certain foods, which can be easily misinterpreted as addiction. As you give yourself permission, notice whether you begin to eat freely, not at or in reaction to imposed limitations. Keep track of experiments with habituation in your journal and build your own case against both restriction and food addiction.

Understanding the concept of habituation is a great start. But the magic happens when the concept becomes embodied, and you feel it for yourself. Mindfulness supports you to venture into this uncharted territory with gentleness, to notice subtle changes between repeated exposures to the same foods, and to observe the gradual arc of foods going from exceptional and potentially dangerous to ordinary and enjoyable when specifically desired.

Eventually, you will notice the foods you thought you *always* wanted are desired only sometimes. And the foods you thought you would eat until they were gone start to linger in the freezer and cabinets for weeks or even months. Trust and have patience.

MINDFUL MOMENT: Begin to Experiment with Habituation

Grab that journal again. What food could you experiment with right now? It may not be the most "charged" food but something more moderate. Once you decide, be sure to have enough of it at home to avoid the risk of scarcity. For example, if you want to experiment with ice cream, have three pints in the freezer at all times. If you finish one, replace it. This reinforces a secure supply, removing the threat of deprivation. Without that stressor to act against, you can eat according to your actual needs and wants—specifically, the amount that allows you to feel you have had *enough*.

Notice your desire for the food. How would you rate it on a scale of 1 to 10 with 1 being "I have no desire for this food" and 10 being "I have high desire for this food"? What sensations, emotions, and thoughts tell you this is the right number? As you eat, check in and rate your desire for the food. Notice whether desire to eat the food coincides with or conflicts with the pleasure you are deriving from it. Repeat this experiment every time the desire for this food arises and notice the trend over repeated exposures.

Sensory-Specific Satiety

Different from habituation, which happens over time with repeated food exposure, sensory-specific satiety occurs within a single eating experience. Continuing to expose your taste buds to the same experience is initially pleasant and rewarding and then eventually diminishes.

My high school economics teacher taught me about sensory-specific satiety by describing the law of diminishing returns. The example he used was pizza. The first slice—magic. The second—still pretty good. The third—okay, this is starting to get old. The fourth—now I'm just going through the motions.

Sometimes called "taste satisfaction," sensory-specific satiety can be recognized by paying mindful attention during an eating experience. Tuning in to subjective enjoyment at the beginning of an eating experience, toward the middle, and as it comes to an end helps you observe these diminishing returns. Again, your "knowing" what is happening may be difficult to describe in words, but the most important part of recognizing and responding to sensory-specific satiety is your capacity to feel it.

Mindfulness not only supports you to recognize sensory-specific satiety, but also to respond to it in a timely and precise manner. If you detect your subjective enjoyment is diminishing but continue to eat to chase or amp up your pleasure, you will inevitably end up overfull and confused. If this has happened, it is still a win. Awareness must always precede change. If, on the other hand, you observe the dissolving nature of an eating experience, you might guide yourself to stop eating in this instance, knowing you'll eat again and feel a higher level of subjective enjoyment when you are hungry.

MINDFUL MOMENT: Notice Sensory-Specific Satiety

The next time you eat, get your journal and record your subjective enjoyment at three points in the eating experience: beginning, middle, and end. Notice the "reward factor" of taste and texture and all those unclassifiable qualities of eating at these three points. Assign them a score between 1 and 10, with 1 being the least rewarding and 10 being the most. Note the differences between your actual experience and what you wished your experience was. Recognizing and working with sensory-specific satiety helps you stay present in your real life as opposed to what I call fighting with reality.

Mindfulness, Interoception, and Satisfaction

Understanding the relationship between satisfaction, mindfulness, and interoception helps you be both the feeler and the observer in your relationship with food and your body. Your senses of smell, sight, feeling, taste, and hearing (though we all experience them differently) are how you engage with the world and place you in the present moment. Mindfully connecting with the senses tells you what is happening in your body and environment in real time.

There are three additional senses: proprioception (awareness of the body's movement and position in space), vestibular system (controlling balance and spatial relations), and interoception. Your interoception—sharpened through mindfulness—helps answer the central question: How do I know whether I'm satisfied?

True satisfaction—built upon the foundation of unconditional permission to eat—derives from interoception of both the sensory qualities of foods and how you feel in your body. You are hardwired to find food pleasurable to eat based on various sensory qualities:

- Taste: sweet, salty, sour, bitter, spicy, acidic, umami, bright, bland

- Temperature: hot, cold, cool, warm, room temperature, or a combination of temperatures simultaneously

- Texture: creamy, soupy, chewy, sticky, thick, thin, gooey, crumbly, al dente, crisp and dry like a thin chip, crisp and wet like iceberg lettuce, crunchy and dense like a corn nut, oily, spongy, hard, soft, or a combination of textures simultaneously

- Sustaining capacity: light, airy, heavy, dense

Sensory characteristics of foods create a unique satisfaction profile. They influence how much of the food you need to reach that undefinable point of enough. They also influence how nurtured you feel in terms of your food choices.

MINDFUL MOMENT: What Sensory Qualities Contribute to Satisfaction for You?

Grab your journal and consider what sensory characteristics contribute to satisfaction. In the left-hand column, write your favorite foods. To the right, write down each food's sensory characteristics. To the right of that, note additional variables that make the food satisfying, such as season, time of day, location, connection with a memory, and so on. Here's an example:

Favorite Foods	Sensory Characteristics	Additional Variables That Make the Food Satisfying
Matzoh ball soup	Warm, different textures of the matzoh balls, carrots, and noodles	Particularly when it's cold out, around the holidays, or when I'm sick
Chubby Hubby ice cream	Combination of creamy ice cream and crunchy chocolate-covered pretzels	Reminds me of being at the beach when I was a kid

Cold pizza	Love the dense "bite" of cold pizza the next morning, the combination of the hard cheese and the slightly acidic, slightly sweet sauce	Feels like I'm back in college reminiscing about a party the night before with my girlfriends

In addition to the sensory characteristics of foods, satisfaction comes through bodily sensations. Usually it is not a single sensation but a constellation of them that signals satisfaction. "Tells" for satisfaction may include:

- *Fullness:* Satisfaction may correlate with fullness when eating foods you like in response to physical hunger. Reaching "comfortable fullness" signals your body is reaching satiety and, because you chose foods that meet your unique preferences, it feels safe and secure to stop there.

- *Taste satisfaction:* Sensory-specific satiety communicates the point at which intensely rewarding foods begin to taste a little less spectacular. Reaching taste satisfaction depends on how hungry you were when you started eating, how novel the food is in terms of your habituation to it, and the circumstances in which you find yourself. Mindful awareness helps you understand continuing to eat after this point won't recapture the satisfaction of the earlier part of the meal, so you can let the eating experience naturally dissolve.

- *Relaxation response:* Many people feel their body relax when they meet both their physiologic needs for calories and macronutrients and their emotional needs for enjoyable foods. Tension may drop away from your jaw, shoulders, chest, back, and belly and you may experience a decreased urgency to keep eating.

- *Spacious mind:* You become preoccupied with food when you are hungry and/or feeling restricted, so your thoughts are free to roam elsewhere when your physical and emotional needs have been met.

- *Feeling of well-being:* By reinforcing unconditional permission to eat, you can choose foods that not only taste good but also feel good in your body. Described as body-food congruence, this awareness comes about later in the process for many. To reach the point of exploring body-food congruence, you must have made peace with food and be willing to pay attention to how eating different foods and quantities of foods makes you feel afterward. I place it here because it is a component of satisfaction, but please wait until you are ready to prioritize this aspect of Intuitive Eating.

MINDFUL MOMENT: What Sensations Communicate Satisfaction?

Come back to your journal to explore the sensations that communicate your body is satisfied:

- What sensations arise when you eat what you want?
- How do your thoughts and feelings change when you give yourself unconditional permission to eat?
- How do you *know* you are satisfied?

How Would You Eat If Satisfaction Were the Goal?

When you are not chronically underfed—both in the quantity of food and the types of foods you are permitted—you are free. Your body is free to experiment with different tastes, textures, temperatures, and smells, to discover which are appealing, and to notice what feels good to eat. Your mind is free to connect with memories and associations. When you are adequately fed, you can discover what you truly like and what works for you.

As your understanding of satisfaction deepens, it becomes more nuanced. Intuitive Eating becomes truly yours. Some of those formerly forbidden fruits might be your favorites, while others lose their shine. Initially, satisfaction might come from not controlling the quantity of food you eat, but eventually, when you realize you can always choose to eat more, eating "enough" actually enhances your pleasure.

MINDFUL MOMENT: Centering Satisfaction

Get your journal and find a restful, uplifted posture. Settle the body by taking three deep breaths, bringing your mind's attention to the feeling of the breath coming in and going out. Ask yourself what, when, how much, and where you would eat if satisfaction were the goal.

- *What:*
    - What types of foods are the most satisfying to you?
    - What are the tastes, textures, temperatures, and sustaining capacities that provide the most satisfaction?
    - Do you prefer little tastes of different things or a larger portion of a single food to enjoy?
    - What do you find uniquely satisfying that others don't?
- *When:*
    - When do you prefer to eat your meals and snacks?
    - How do your unique preferences align with or diverge from common meal and snack times?
- *How much:*
    - What degree of fullness aligns with satisfaction for you?
    - Are fewer, larger meals more satisfying? More frequent, smaller meals?
- *Where:*
    - What is your preferred environment to eat?
    - What room temperature do you like? Lighting? Location? Seating arrangement?
    - Are there environmental factors that are important for you to avoid to enhance satisfaction?

Disappointing Eating Experiences

Not every eating experience will be stellar. Recipes don't come out as planned, your favorite restaurant can have an off night, and takeout is rarely what you imagine. You won't always reach satisfaction even when you prioritize it.

When you center satisfaction, you might have an unspoken wish that every meal and snack meet your highest expectations. It is wonderful to prize true satisfaction and to discern your preferences as they change moment to moment, meal to meal, day to day.

Eventually and inevitably, though, something will fail to meet your expectations. You won't like it, but with mindfulness, a disappointing meal can be illuminating. You might notice, for example, that when the quality of the food isn't great, you compensate with greater quantity. You might notice prolonged preoccupation with food, even after eating is over. All of this is completely normal. The noticing is valuable.

Recognizing and dealing with disappointing eating experiences is one way to directly and intentionally confront discomfort, sadness, and that icky feeling of unsatisfactoriness. First noble truth alert! This is also a great way to get comfortable with discomfort. Experiment with discomfort as it relates to food first and eventually as it relates to life in general.

Recognizing dissatisfaction in eating is living your actual life: the life that is sometimes not what you want. Feeling, allowing, and being with dissatisfaction has the potential to heighten true satisfaction when it spontaneously arises.

MINDFUL MOMENT: Dealing with Disappointment

The next time you have a disappointing eating experience, grab your journal and notice the gap between expectations and reality. What were you hoping for in terms of taste, texture, temperature, sustaining capacity, other sensory characteristics? Where did the food or eating experience fall short? At what point did you recognize this? How did you respond physically? How did you respond emotionally? How did you speak to yourself? What, if any, ripple effects did the disappointing eating experience have in your day and/or on your subsequent eating experiences?

MINDFUL MOMENT: The Next Best Thing

Here you will explore prioritizing satisfaction when your first choice is not available. Grab your journal. Write down a food you crave occasionally. What do you enjoy most about it? What specific tastes, textures, temperatures, and sustaining capacities appeal to you? Where do you get the best version of this food, the one you love the most?

Imagine you're craving that food, but for some reason you cannot get it. What is the most important characteristic of that food in this moment? What other foods possess that important characteristic? A couple of examples can be found below.

Original Craving	Most Important Characteristic	Next Best Thing(s)
Pizza from your favorite pizzeria	Acidic sweetness of the tomato sauce	Pasta with tomato sauce, chips and salsa, tomato soup
	The gooiness of the cheese	Grilled cheese, panino, calzone, baked ziti
	The chewiness of the crust	Sandwich on a baguette, soft pretzel, bagel with cream cheese
Vietnamese pho	Warm broth	Chicken noodle soup, another kind of brothy soup, bone broth
	Aromatic spices	Five-spice tofu, quick-cook ramen, a special aromatic tea
	Combination of temperatures and textures	Grain bowl with cool greens and warm grains, burrito with hot and cold ingredients, tacos

The more attention you pay to the specific characteristics that satisfy, the more equipped you are to meet your needs, even when you can't have exactly what you want.

I can't help but wonder what our society would look like if we all centered satisfaction. A few things I predict: SnackWell's would never have existed. Neither would 100-calorie packs of anything or food companies that make calorie-controlled meals or modified foods containing unnaturally low amounts of carbs or fats. Food scales and measuring cups would be reserved for bakers. Food-centered holidays like Halloween, Christmas, Ramadan, and Passover would be enjoyed and not feared. Gym memberships would remain fairly consistent throughout the year, not peaking right after New Year's or before the summer months.

I imagine binge-eating rates would drop dramatically without the physical and emotional restriction necessary to drive binge behavior. Perhaps people would spend money on things that enhance their quality of life, like books, travel, and charitable donations, rather than on diet foods and programs. Healthy cookbooks would focus on both the experience of eating and how you feel as the result of eating certain foods.

I think we would be happier, clearer about our wants and needs, and better able to care for ourselves. We would trust our bodies and feel confident in our judgment as the experts of ourselves.

What Can You Celebrate?

- What knowledge did you confirm?

- What do you understand now about your relationship with satisfaction that you didn't before?

- What are you excited to pay attention to?

CHAPTER 6

Movement

Your body was made to move. It is part of what makes you human. When you were a baby, you moved however felt right to you in the moment: snuggling, rolling over, crawling, walking, running, jumping, skipping, dancing. You weren't consciously aware of how your body wanted to move. You just moved!

If you can't remember feeling born to move, just watch a child. See what happens when you release them on a playground, soccer field, or dance floor. There is joy, concentration, and adaptation. No shame or self-doubt. Not right away, at least. The desire to move your body doesn't just go away. It may go underground, but it's still there. Fortunately, Intuitive Eating and mindfulness pave the way to rediscover movement. Your way.

Depending on your ability or relationship with chronic illness or pain, your body craves movement. Your relationship with movement—marketed as exercise, working out, or calorie burning—has likely been distorted by diet culture. According to diet culture, moving your body is an obligation that earns you the right to eat, to take up space, to even exist. It's something you must do, rather than something you choose to do. It's a means to an end rather than something done for the experience itself.

Remember, you are the expert of yourself. No one can tell you what to do! Removing rules and judgments around eating ultimately helps you make peace with food, and removing rules and judgments around movement liberates you to discover how you want to move. And just as you crave a variety of foods when you give yourself full and unconditional permission to eat, you crave different types of movement when it's something you choose to do.

Your body enjoys a range of movement. You can sense and respond to your desire for movement just as you can sense and respond to your desire for certain eating experiences. Like self-regulating what and when and how much you eat, your body senses, interprets, and responds to the desire for movement. There may be work to do, but you will get there.

That work begins by understanding how diet culture harmed your relationship with movement. Learning some basic facts about your body and movement helps you separate the movement you *choose* to do from the exercise you were told you *had* to do. Healing your relationship with movement comes through experimentation and data collection, ultimately helping you redefine what movement means for you.[15] First, let's explore associations.

MINDFUL MOMENT: Separate the Idea of Exercise from Movement

Grab your journal and explore associations with the word "exercise":

- What does "exercise" bring to mind?

- When do you first remember hearing about exercising for weight control?

- Who did you hear it from and what was their relationship to you?

- Who were exercise "influencers" at the time? How did that impact your interpretation?

- How did you feel about "obligatory exercise"? Were you happy for the clear prescription? Did you rebel and distance yourself from exercise?

- How did your relationship with exercise evolve over time? What were the major phases?

Now consider the word "movement":

- What images arise when you hear the word "movement"?

- What thoughts and feelings arise?

- How are they similar or different from your response to the word "exercise"?

- How do you feel about the suggestion that movement is different from exercise? Suspicious? Anxious? Hopeful?

Please remember that this part of your Intuitive Eating journey, too, will unfold naturally. There is no rush. Your new relationship with movement will continue to evolve for the rest of your life. One thing remains true: you have your hand on the dial. And mindfulness supports you to sense and respond to your changing needs.

Diet Culture Distorted Your Relationship with Movement

Before attempting to heal your relationship with movement, it is useful to understand where it went wrong. The diet culture's messages about movement likely overshadowed moving your body because it was enjoyable.

Diet culture might have harmed your relationship with movement in many ways: telling you to do unpleasant exercise to reap desirable outcomes; bullying you to work out for longer than you want to maximize calories burned or muscle fatigue achieved; encouraging you to disconnect from your body to get through exercise, distracting yourself through it or focusing on how you'll feel afterward. All of these could alienate you from any internal desire to move.

When I studied nutrition, I mostly learned about exercise as a way to keep body weight in check. The "eat less, move more" approach implicitly suggested you eat too much and don't move your body enough. Exercise was a way to "stay on track," earn your calories, and (I often felt) justify your existence.

Exercise could also change your body's appearance. Cardiovascular exercise burned calories, while strength training built and toned muscle. Over time, certain types of exercise rose and fell in popularity, but these two basic concepts remained. Whether burning calories or sculpting the body's surface, the emphasis was on appearance. This emphasis on outcome inherently conflicts with mindfulness, which highlights present-moment awareness.

No pain, no gain. Suffer now, you'll thank yourself later. Do whatever is necessary to achieve the outcome of thinness, weight loss, a lifted derriere, six-pack abs, and so on. Focusing on the end point seriously impacts your capacity for presence and connection with your embodied experience of movement. This may have caused you to go through the motions, exercise on autopilot, and check out when moving. Or it may have provoked avoidance, rebellion, and resignation.

MINDFUL MOMENT: Explore Your Childhood Relationship with Movement

In your journal, explore your relationship with movement as a child. Before you thought about moving your body to burn calories, what did you love to do? Swing on the swings? Climb on the monkey bars? Run races? Jump waves? Did you love to bicycle or speed on a scooter? Or lie on your back resting and looking up into the trees?

Can you remember enjoying moving your body in specific ways? Was it vigorous, rhythmic, fast, or slow? Did you get out of breath or was it something you could keep up for long periods of time? Can you reconnect with the part of you that *knew* you wanted to move that way? How does it feel to recognize there was an intelligent body that knew how it wanted to move?

You're not trying to go back in time and recapture anything, but it can be helpful to reconnect with a younger you to understand what has changed and to recall a less complicated time. If, after doing this exercise, memories emerge about early associations with movement, capture them in your journal.

Some Truths About Movement

Your body is synonymous with movement. Even when perfectly still, your body is in constant motion. The breath is coming in and going out. Blood is coursing through your veins. Tiny neurons are firing. Tissues are continuously remodeled as cells die and are replaced. This has several implications.

You Don't Need to Earn Your Calories

Most of your calorie needs go toward what is known as basal metabolic rate (BMR), which is the amount of energy consumed by your body at rest. One method of estimating energy needs adds an "activity factor," which is usually a moderate addition to our baseline needs. This means movement is not necessary to earn the right to eat.

Here's an example. A body that requires 2,500 calories to operate at rest might require an additional 500 to 750 calories with a moderate amount of activity. If that same person were to restrict intake on days they weren't doing physical activity, they risk shorting their body's needs. Done regularly, the body's compensatory mechanisms might kick in to fight perceived starvation. Over time, metabolism could slow down, physical performance could suffer, and someone cutting calories in this way is likely to feel very confused.

The best way to approach nourishing your body remains the same:

- Focus on internal sensations of hunger, fullness, satisfaction, and personal preference

- Feed yourself regularly throughout the day with a balance of protein, carbohydrate, and fat

- Stay flexible because no two days have identical energy needs and your body can adapt to day-to-day variability

Movement Exists on Multiple Spectrums

How you move your body—like hunger and fullness and many other things—exists on multiple spectrums: intensity, solo to group, environment, fitness level required, and other considerations such as disability, injury, chronic pain, or other differences. One such spectrum is intensity; physical activity ranges from stillness to vigorous. When at rest, heart and breathing rates slow, with moderate activity they speed up, and when moving energetically even more so. Consider viewing movement this way as you cultivate a new relationship with it.

Here are some examples of movement across the spectrum of intensity. Many of these could fit in multiple categories and be adjusted in terms of intensity:

- *Stillness:* meditating, savasana, body scan, napping, daydreaming, people watching, rest

- *Gentle:* stretching, slow flow yoga, restorative yoga, yin yoga, gardening, bowling, golf, active rest, ping pong, badminton, aqua aerobics, miniature golf, running errands, slow walking

- *Precise:* Pilates, Iyengar yoga, strength training, ballet, stand up paddleboard, mindful walking

- *Sensual:* pole dancing, Zumba, salsa, tango, 5Rhythms, Nia, Gyrotonic, sex, masturbation

- *Moderate:* bicycling, fast walking, swimming, treading water, raking leaves, shoveling snow, ice skating, roller skating, hip-hop dancing, martial arts, ballroom dancing, playing with kids, sailing

- *Vigorous:* ashtanga yoga, running, elliptical, hiking, rowing, rock climbing, racquetball, tennis, kickboxing, aerobics, HIIT, downhill skiing, cross-country skiing, team sports like basketball or soccer

Different movement intensities might appeal to your nervous system at different times. Other spectrums on which movement exists include with whom you do it, the environment in which you do it, and the fitness level required to begin. The point here is to expand how you think of movement. As you would consider the sensory characteristics of foods, consider the sensory characteristics of different kinds of movement. Do you like to move your body alone, with one other person, or with a small or large group? What kind of environment feels safest, most accessible, and inviting? Indoor or outdoor, warm or cool or cold weather, around or away from other people, in the morning or daytime or evening?

Disability, injuries, chronic pain, health conditions, cardiorespiratory fitness, and conditioning levels when you begin a certain type of movement also matter. Please consult with your health care provider before beginning any type of movement. You might also consult an exercise physiologist, physical trainer, or articles from a reliable source for how to approach it.

Michele's Story

Michele was an avid downhill skier but started to experience a lot of knee pain. She was convinced her pain was caused by "all the excess weight I'm carrying around." We discussed both the factual and the emotional aspects of this experience. Key facts included the similar incidence of knee pain among individuals in larger and smaller bodies and her family history of degenerative joint disease independent of weight. The idea her pain wasn't the result of anything Michele had done wrong took time to sink in. She agreed to explore physical therapy, acupuncture, targeted weight training to strengthen the knee area, meditation, stress relief, and prioritizing sleep, all of which can mitigate the subjective experience of pain.

Michele discovered that not moving her body because she felt badly about it worsened her pain. She permitted herself to mourn the loss of skiing and acknowledged the difficulty in getting older and having her body change. She also started cross-country skiing, which was easier on her joints.

Enjoyable and Sustainable Movement Makes You Happier and Healthier

Put simply: movement makes you happier and healthier without any connection with weight.[16] Minus all the complexity around movement, most of us discover we want to move in different ways. The diet culture creates false standards about what "counts" as movement, but realistically, what you do every day, from the most subtle kinds of movement to more energetic ones, affects your body metabolically, physiologically, and even psychologically.

A psychiatrist once said that movement is the most underused non-pharmacologic antidepressant. Hyperbole aside, the benefits of movement are undeniable. Improved blood sugar control, insulin sensitivity, cholesterol, liver function, sleep, pain management, and bone density and decreased depression and anxiety are just a few of the health benefits observed in studies on movement. And more studies are showing that a weight-neutral approach to movement in which increasing cardiorespiratory fitness and physical activity is encouraged independent of emphasis on weight loss reduces death rate more than intentional weight loss in people in larger bodies.

MINDFUL MOMENT: Movement Contemplation

Sit or lie down in a comfortable position. Find a balance between restful and uplifted so your body feels alert. Your eyes can be closed or gently open. Take a few minutes to feel your breath, focusing your mind's attention on the sensations of breath in and out through the nose.

Bring the following questions to mind:

- What intensity of movement appeals to me right now?

- How do I want to feel as I engage in movement?

- How does my body want to move?

- What parts of my body want to move?

- Who do I want to be with when I move my body?

- Do I want to be hot, warm, cool, or even cold? Inside or outside?

- What time of day feels most appealing?

- What other considerations are important to me, such as season, outdoor temperature, health conditions, cardiorespiratory fitness level, or injury?

Capture "noticings" in your journal. Return to this exercise as the seasons change, as your fitness level changes, as you age, and any time you wish to consult your body regarding movement.

Helene's Story

Helene was a dancer all her life. She loved feeling "in her body," yet her body caused her suffering because of how it had changed when she gained weight. Surrounded by other dancers, Helene had trouble accepting her body. She even questioned why her adult students came to learn from her, suggesting she felt she had nothing to offer if she didn't live in a "dancer's body." We discussed the sadness, anger, and confusion inherent in living in a culture that teaches you to hate your body, and we focused on dropping into her body and inquiring as to what types of movement she wanted to do.

Helene realized she had several distinct ways in which she wanted to move, for example, exercising so vigorously she felt she was "hunting buffalo on the plain" so she could take a cold shower and fall into bed exhausted. Helene discovered she always had her hand on the dial regarding the pace, intensity, and duration of movement so it fit her specific needs in the moment. Eventually, she realized she offered her students something unique: a dance teacher in a regular body who inspired everyone to pursue their love of dance.

When Are You Ready to Engage with Movement?

Similar to fullness, movement requires care when approaching it. As you recall, I suggested you leave fullness until stopping eating at a point that feels like "enough" is not obligatory but a form of compassionate self-care—one that even enhances pleasure. For that same reason, reframing movement may come later for you, and that is completely normal and fine.

You are ready to engage with movement when your body tells you it wants to move, and when moving in different ways feels like a means of caring for your body and tending to its ever-changing needs. Some examples of approaching movement in this way might include:

- Tending to physical pain

- Loosening muscle and joint tightness

- Increasing range of motion

- Addressing general fatigue

- Feeling more engaged in your surroundings

- Releasing physical and emotional tension

- Expressing your response to music

- Breaking out of inertia and doing *something* different

- Wanting to feel something different

- Desiring a feeling of exhilaration

- Wanting to "get your heart pumping"

- Sharing an activity with someone

When you decide to engage with movement, remember to pay attention to the in-the-moment process. On how you feel inside rather than how you appear to others. Feeling into your body and being with yourself while moving rather than focusing on how you will look as the result of moving your body. Mindfulness shows you the way: place your awareness on the sensations of whatever movement you're engaged in and when attention strays and you become absorbed in thought, gently guide it back to your present-moment body.

If diet mentality creeps in—which it is bound to do because you still live in this culture—don't panic. Acknowledge this is a process of unlearning and reframing according to your own values. Remember that you have been immersed in diet culture far longer than you have been practicing Intuitive Eating. And remember that the complexity of your relationship with movement is not uniquely yours (bringing movement back into your life, however, will be uniquely yours). Then celebrate the progress you've already made even if it is simply a willingness to see things differently.

If you experiment with movement and any of the following arises, it might still be premature:

- Intense shame and resistance around moving

- A trajectory in which you feel the need to do more and more

- Falling back into habits of weighing movement and food intake

- Consistently putting off movement

- Not carrying out your own plans to do some form of movement

- Waiting for "perfect conditions" to move your body

Redefine and Reclaim Movement for Yourself

A movement practice should feel like your own: directly related to who you are, how you feel, and what you need in the present moment and in a grander way. It may even draw on your history with "exercise" by healing specific wounds and reclaiming a form of movement that was distorted by diet mentality.

Mindfulness Helps You Know

Remember mindfulness happens in your body. You are not attempting to transcend the body. Without the body, there is no mindfulness practice. Without the body, there is no joy of movement. The body is the vehicle for waking up to the nature of reality, the instrument with which you interact with the world.

Remember one of those key questions you learned in chapter 1: "How do I know?" Trusting your body and your judgment as it navigates this part of your Intuitive Eating path has everything to do with the answer to that question. Knowing happens in the body.

MINDFUL MOMENT: Bedtime Body Awareness

Do this practice when you get into bed at night.

1. As you lie down, notice sensations. Just feel them at first, resisting the desire to attach a judgment of positive, negative, or neutral.

2. Next, notice the firmness of the mattress beneath you. The pillow under your head. The texture of the clothing or sheets touching your skin. Notice the weight of the blankets on top of you. What are your preferences? How close are these sensations to your preferences? For example, is the firmness of the mattress just right? Too soft? Too hard? How do you know?

3. Then get into a position that feels comfortable to fall asleep. Is that on the left side? The right side? On your back? Stomach? How do you know this is the position your body wants to be in? What specifically tells you this is "right" for right now?

4. As you drift into twilight between sleeping and waking, what is it like to *know* what feels right for your body in this moment? How does it feel to be the only person who could possibly know what is right for your body?

MINDFUL MOMENT: Mindful Walking

Practice mindful walking whenever you are waiting somewhere, before or after another form of movement, or even in your home. The object of your attention is the sensation of your foot on the ground.

1. In the first stage, notice yourself stepping, stepping, stepping. Feel the heel come down, roll through the middle of the foot to the toe, and push off the ball and toes. If your mind wanders, notice, release whatever thought distracted you, and redirect your attention back to the sensation of your foot on the ground.

2. In the second stage, become aware of how at the end of one step, your body shifts to take the next step.

3. In the third stage, notice stepping, shifting, and picking up. Stepping, shifting, and picking up.

The degree of mindfulness and progression shared in this practice can be applied to any form of movement.

Constancy over Consistency

One of the myths about movement is that it must look the same every day, every week, every year. The concept of consistency has halted many a movement plan before it ever started. If you imagine going from never moving to moving every day, you could be overwhelmed. There is no need for that. Rather than consistency, could you allow your relationship to movement to be constant? Could you commit to a constant intention to move your body as your body wishes. Your body is always changing, healing, and responding to different events and environments, so its need for movement will always be different. It's fine to do the same thing day to day, but it's also wonderful to allow your movement practice to be responsive to changing needs. Ask yourself, *How do I want to move my body today?*

Summon Self-Compassion

The process of redefining and reclaiming movement—of developing a practice of listening to your body and responding to its needs—lasts a lifetime. What if the background noise for this redefinition could be self-compassionate rather than self-aggressive?

A simple three-step self-compassion formula could be applied to any part of your Intuitive Eating path, including movement. Whenever you encounter challenges, rouse self-compassion by:

1. Acknowledging suffering

2. Normalizing your experience

3. Offering yourself kindness

If you feel winded as you build greater cardiorespiratory fitness, you might say to yourself: *This is hard, I haven't moved my body in this way in a while and it needs to catch up. My automatic reaction is to be hard on myself, but every body needs to come up to speed when it starts a new movement practice. The best I can do is continue fueling my body, meet its basic needs, and take breaks when I need to so I can start again.*

If your belly gets in your way as you do a forward bend in yoga, you might say: *It's so hard to move when it feels like my body doesn't cooperate. The diet culture says there is a specific body for yoga and my body isn't like that. But every body deserves to move and to feel the benefits of movement. I can acknowledge this difficulty and keep connecting with my body through yoga.*

If you feel pain doing the type of movement you wish to do, you might say: *I want to blame my body size for feeling this pain, but that is not the only reason bodies feel pain. It is normal for all bodies to feel pain sometimes. I will find a form of movement that feels good to me and I will tend to my pain by resting, comforting, and strengthening my body so it can continue to move.*

Reclaiming movement is a radical act in a world still dominated by diet culture. Just imagine what the world would feel like if we were to listen and respond to our bodies. What would it be like if all bodies were accorded the same right to respect, care, love, attention, pleasure, well-being, and inclusion? Not in spite of our differences, but in full view of them.

Mindfulness and Intuitive Eating begin and end with the body. Engaging with your hunger, fullness, satisfaction, and movement helps you maintain a connection with these practices as they unfold for the rest of your life.

What Can You Celebrate?

- What did you recall about early experiences with movement?

- What textures of movement are appealing to your nervous system?

- What are you excited about trying?

- Do you feel ready to explore movement? Why or why not?

PART II

Mindfulness of Feelings

Mindfulness of feelings is the willingness to feel what is happening in your body and in your heart—and to stay. It is allowing things (and yourself) to be as they are and holding your seat.

Building upon the foundation of mindfulness of the body—because you have stabilized the body by unconditionally meeting its needs—you become able to tolerate, open, and soften toward the full range of your emotions.

Mindfulness of feelings is not separate from the body, where true healing happens. Your nervous system is always working to protect you—perceiving signs of safety and danger. Interoception—honed through mindfulness of body—allows this unconscious perception to be recognized, interpreted, and responded to consciously, with kindness.

CHAPTER 7

The Biology of Emotion

We are emotional beings. And that is a wonderful thing. Don't let anyone tell you otherwise.

I debate this topic with my partner, who is a scientist and very rational. He believes in logic: people make decisions objectively by assessing the data, and therefore rational thought drives behavior. I believe the opposite: emotions rule the world. Whether trends in the stock market, the decision to buy a certain pair of shoes or brand of cereal, or what movie to watch, feelings are running the show.

What will make me feel how I want to feel? What will help me avoid what I don't want to feel? What feels like "me"? What makes me feel like the person I want to be? What can I do to feel good? And what can I do to avoid feeling bad? These are the questions you probably unconsciously ask yourself throughout the day. And they drive how you think and act.

Even though you are inherently emotional and experience many feelings a day, you may not feel particularly well equipped to deal with the full range of your emotions. You might have an oversimplified understanding of them—you are either happy or sad, agreeable or angry, full or empty. You might think only "positive" emotions are valuable, while the so-called "negative" ones should be eliminated. If you have a feeling you like, you want to hold on to it. If you have one that makes you uncomfortable, you might feel threatened, scared, and confused, and want to get rid of it pronto.

Add food and body to this mix and things get interesting. Eating, dieting, weight, and movement are all emotional. None of this is a problem. Neither is not knowing how to work with strong emotions yet. Most of us never learn this or have it modeled for us.

This chapter contains some broad strokes about your emotions—the full spectrum of your emotions. You'll see how your feelings about your feelings affect, well, your feelings. And you'll begin to experiment with feeling your emotions more directly—without adding anything or taking anything away—with the help of mindfulness and compassion.

But First, a Note About Trauma

The Buddhist tradition encourages people to lean into their emotional discomfort. "Take it to the meditation cushion" is a common response when people experience painful feelings. Leaning into the discomfort is a wonderful suggestion, but only if your nervous system can tolerate it. Not everyone's nervous system can always tolerate all kinds of discomfort. The key is discerning the discomfort that is safe to lean into and the discomfort to respectfully back away from, at least for now.

Mindfulness is meant to relieve suffering. But if you have trauma, whether you experienced a single traumatic event or multiple or repeated events, mindfulness might paradoxically intensify your suffering by amplifying unprocessed energy in the body.[17] If you know you have trauma, it's best to speak to a mental health clinician before beginning a meditation practice or practicing mindfulness. Particularly if your clinician is trauma-sensitive, they can help you know whether and when your body and mind are ready for such practices.

Sometimes you can't know how you will react to a mindfulness practice. If you begin to meditate or practice mindfulness and something feels "off," stop meditating, and come back into the present moment by naming five objects you can see and touch—for example, orange blanket, painting of trees, white couch, yellow diary, green glass. When you can, consult with someone who is informed about trauma, mindfulness, and the nervous system. Some clues your nervous system might not be ready for the stillness and focused attention of mindfulness include:

- Hyperarousal: anxious, tense, overwhelmed, feeling out of control, angry, irritable, wanting to run away

- Hypoarousal: collapsed, sleepy, numb, frozen, spacey, shut down, zoned out

If you have experienced trauma, do not despair. You can still be an Intuitive Eater, and likely will be able to complement that with mindfulness somehow. The beauty of recognizing exactly where you are and what you need is that you work with reality, which is the ultimate point of meditation! That reality might be your nervous system needs some TLC before it can pay such close attention to emotions and physical states. The following resources elegantly address the nuanced needs of people with trauma:

- *Trauma-Sensitive Mindfulness: Practices for Safe and Transformative Healing* by David Treleaven, 2018

- *Restorative Yoga for Ethnic and Race-Based Stress and Trauma* by Gail Parker, 2020

- *Transforming Ethnic and Race-Based Traumatic Stress with Yoga* by Gail Parker, 2021

- *The Body Keeps the Score: Brain, Mind, and Body in the Healing of Trauma* by Bessel van der Kolk, 2015

The Emotional Landscape

When I envision my feelings, I see the positive ones—happiness, joy, contentment, satisfaction, gratitude, curiosity, playfulness, and others—above an imaginary horizon. Negative emotions like sadness, anger, jealousy, and loneliness, on the other hand, lie below.

I used to try to live only in the space above the horizon. When I did feel good, however, I only enjoyed that briefly before I worried about how I was going to stay there. More often than not, positive emotions felt very precarious and, rather than savoring them, I felt anxious about losing them.

Uncomfortable emotions also felt impossible to stay with. Not only did I feel the discomfort and pain of the core emotion, but I also amplified my suffering by feeling badly about feeling badly. If I felt lonely, for example, I couldn't just feel pure loneliness. Instead, shame about feeling lonely took over, compounding my suffering.

More recently I learned to value all of my emotions—the good, the bad, and everything in between. That awareness was hard won after realizing how judgments about my emotions distorted my capacity to experience my life directly. When I anxiously grasped onto positive emotions for fear of losing them, when I felt terrible for feeling terrible, I was not giving myself a chance to feel the original emotions. I was so quick to try to manage and control them, I robbed myself of my real experience. This cost me dearly.

Meditation and mindfulness gave me the tools to stay with my in-the-moment self, and to experience what is arising in a pure, undistorted way. It's not that I always like what I'm experiencing, but at least I know it's real.

When I look at the horizon image with the "positive" emotions above and the "negative" ones below, I don't judge some as better than others. Some are subjectively more pleasant, but they all have value, and feeling them—wholly and directly—adds richness to my life.

The Feelings Wheel

Different sources have tried to capture the spectrum of feelings visually. My favorite was created by Australian pastor Geoffrey Roberts. I love it not because it is the be-all and end-all, but because it provides language and a framework to describe what is rarely verbalized.

Roberts presented seven core emotions—happy, surprised, sad, bad, angry, disgusted, and fearful. This core is surrounded by two concentric circles: the seven emotions are first dissected into 41 more specific feelings, and then those 41 are further divided into 82 for a total of 130 separate feelings. Happy, for example, has nine subdivisions: playful, content, interested, proud, accepted, powerful, peaceful, trusting, and optimistic. There's a subtle but important difference between feeling happy and feeling proud, which can be further distinguished into successful or confident. Sad, on the other hand, encompasses lonely, vulnerable, despair, guilty, depressed, or hurt. There is power in clarifying that, more than sad, you feel vulnerable, and even more specifically you feel either victimized or fragile. To learn more about this version of the Feelings Wheel, visit https://feelingswheel.com.

The Feelings Wheel encourages you to dig deeper and fine-tune how you describe your internal environment. It helps you know yourself and each of your emotions—even if they are fleeting—with greater precision. Am I sad or am I feeling powerless? Am I angry or feeling disrespected? Getting this granular with your own experience—paying yourself this level of compassionate attention—helps you know yourself better.

In chapter 2, you learned about polyvagal theory, a framework for understanding your nervous system, how it protects you, and what it feels like in your body when regulated (feeling safe and connected in the ventral state) and when dysregulated (whether angry or anxious in the fight-or-flight sympathetic state or shutdown and collapsed in the dorsal state). Based on this understanding of how your biology responds to different situations, you can "notice and name." When you notice and name what is happening in your nervous system, you are both experiencing your emotion in real time and bringing it into focus rather than letting it remain hazy and unknown. Noticing and naming what is happening in real time allows you to work with emotion.

MINDFUL MOMENT: Notice and Name

Get your journal and create a page called "Notice and Name." For one week, set an alarm to go off four times during the day—morning, noon, afternoon, and night. When it sounds, take a moment to notice and name what you are feeling.

Each time, begin by closing your eyes (or leaving them gently open) and taking three deep breaths, focusing your attention on the feeling of the breath coming in and going out through the nose. After three breaths, inquire inward to determine how you are feeling. If, when you ask yourself, the response is happy or sad, for example, could you go deeper? Be more specific?

Use the Feelings Wheel to identify a more precise word for what you are feeling at these four points in the day. You may also do this exercise when a particular feeling strikes you—either pleasantly or unpleasantly. Notice and give a name to what is happening right then and there. If you don't notice anything, that's okay too. Inquiring inward creates a practice that takes root, eventually revealing useful information about your internal environment.

Noticing and naming takes practice. It won't become automatic overnight. Begin by noticing and naming regularly and intentionally. After several weeks, see if there are times you notice and name without planning to.

Difficult Emotions

You are hardwired to prefer comfort and ease over discomfort and struggle because it protects you. Evolutionarily, suffering was dangerous and potentially life-threatening. Avoiding dangerous situations made survival more likely.

You probably therefore associate positive emotions with safety and negative ones with danger. This is natural and normal. When the relationship with positive emotions becomes desperate, and when negative emotions feel intolerable, things get weird. Buddhist philosophy acknowledges there are emotions we like and those we dislike. That natural preference is fine. When you habitually grasp onto positive feelings and push away negative ones, however, suffering actually increases.

All phenomena follow a predictable life cycle: they arise, level off, and eventually dissolve. While eating an enjoyable meal, for example, pleasure rises, plateaus, and then dissipates. Difficult emotions are no different. Sadness begins by arising, then it reaches a point where it levels off, and ultimately it dissolves. Rising, leveling off, and dissolving may happen over a long arc of time, or it may happen in little bursts, or a combination of the two.

Automatically reacting to negative emotions may distort them and alter that life cycle. The merest hint of a negative emotion can feel so unsafe that, before you notice, you react to avoid that suffering. For example, as a satisfying dinner winds down and the sometimes-onerous routine of kids' bath and bedtime must commence, despair might set in. Your natural aversion to this feeling could elicit an automatic reaction of fear, irritation, confusion, or something else. Rather than feeling the despair, therefore, you compound your discomfort by feeling badly about feeling badly. Feeling badly about feeling badly often leads people to emotionally overeat. Reacting to avoiding feeling despair might also cost you a nuanced experience of bath time and bedtime, like bubble beards and nighttime gratitude practice. The immediate reaction to a strong feeling takes you out of the moment, making it impossible to be with things as they are.

In Buddhist philosophy this is called the suffering of suffering. Some suffering is inevitable in life. You cannot control or sidestep it. What you can control to some degree, however, is the suffering of suffering, including how you react to painful emotions.

MINDFUL MOMENT: How Do You Feel About How You Feel?

This exercise builds on the previous one in which you notice and name emotions. You are invited to notice the cascade of emotions brought about by your original feeling.

As you notice and name emotions that arise throughout the day, see whether you also notice secondary emotions in response to the primary emotion. Feeling lonely could provoke feelings of shame, for example. Also notice whether secondary emotions feel even stronger, scarier, or more painful than the original.

Continue to work with your emotions this way and become familiar with your full spectrum. With patience and practice you might appreciate even "negative" emotions.

Mindfulness and Perception of Safety and Danger

Your nervous system constantly scans for signs of safety and danger in a process called neuroception. Sometimes it assesses a situation as dangerous even if it is not objectively dangerous. The perceptions of the nervous system are conditioned by past experiences. For example, if a parent disapproved every time you wanted dessert, and that disapproval made you feel ashamed, you might feel the humiliating sinking sensation of shame whenever you crave something sweet. Sweets mean danger.

The nervous system perceives safety and danger unconsciously, sometimes before you realize you are reacting. Perceived danger leads to a dysregulated nervous system, which leads to negative feelings, reactive behaviors, and a "story" you concoct about what happened. Building on the scenario above, a story might be: "I'm craving something sweet, but sweets are bad. It's bad to want sweets; desiring sweets can change how people look at me. If I want love and approval, I shouldn't crave sweets and definitely should not give in when I do want them." Alternatively: "I'm craving something sweet, but I can't have them because I'm in a larger body. Other people can eat sweets if they are in smaller bodies, so I can't even think about eating sweets until I lose weight."

Mindfulness helps bring your body's unconscious reactions into the conscious realm. Practicing noticing and naming slows things down enough to avoid an automatic and unwitting emotional domino effect. You see how the desire for sweets leads to that sinking feeling and remember where that leads you.

Becoming more conscious of yourself stabilizes your nervous system, helping it more accurately read the environment. A stabilized nervous system might recognize the following: "I'm craving something sweet. This feels hard because of the messages I received about sweets and my body when I was a child. But when I don't respect my cravings, they get more intense and lead to a binge. I should offer myself compassion and eat what I want with full permission and attention."

In addition to a more accurate perception, you witness the full spectrum of your emotions while holding your seat. You feel sadness and vulnerability for the child who was shamed for wanting an enjoyable eating experience and, in a way, reparent her to have a healthy relationship with sweets.

Emotions Occur in the Body

You might experience emotions as concepts: challenging to pin down, difficult to tolerate, happening in a realm apart from the body. But emotions are not separate from your body. The mind-body connection is evident in how humans feel—literally feel—emotions as bodily sensations. Getting choked up. Feeling a pit in the stomach. Fire in the belly. Skin crawling. These are embodied emotional experiences. The mind-body connection is also essential in how to soothe yourself.

When I delved deeper into this work about ten years ago, my mentor Evelyn Tribole described how every emotion has an associated physical sensation. When I was describing the cascade of events leading up to a client's binge, for example, Evelyn prompted me to inquire what was happening in my client's body, specifically what sensations she was feeling. I took this concept in intellectually but my understanding was more conceptual than embodied.

Seeking to understand my own emotions more deeply—whenever I remembered to inquire within as to what sensations were present—I felt stuck at the bottom of a well. I couldn't climb out or break through the thick walls around me. I quickly gave up, fearing I was not capable of such nuanced awareness. I continued to inquire within, if only briefly, with the hope that I might notice something someday.

A few years later—through meditation, mindfulness practices, and learning about polyvagal theory—I felt my emotions in my body. Anxiety was a buzzy sensation in my lips, tension in my upper stomach, and restlessness in my arms. Feeling emotions in my body, I suddenly understood my strong negative reactions to painful ones: my body felt threatened! And I saw how it was simply trying to protect me from that perceived danger.

Some researchers have attempted to map emotions in the body.[18] Like a heat map, the emotional body map highlights activation (shown in bright or dark hues of red and yellow) and deactivation (shown as black) when emotions are experienced. For example, gratefulness comprises activation in the torso, face, and brain. Despair shows activation in these areas as well as the lower belly.

MINDFUL MOMENT: Feel Emotions in Your Body

You can map sensations associated with emotions in your own body. Get your journal. Pick a time when you are noticing and naming. Inquire inward as to where you can feel your emotion.

Beginning with the bottom of the feet, lightly scan the body. You may notice sensations are pleasant, unpleasant, or neutral. Parts of the body may feel activated, as if there is energy coursing through them with sensations like warmth, tingling, surging, or crawling. Parts of the body may feel deactivated—dormant, heavy, cold, numb, or inanimate.

Notice the texture and temperature of sensations. Notice whether colors or shapes occur to you. Notice whether sensations change with time—rapidly or slowly—as you pay attention. Record your "noticings" in your journal.

You may also do this exercise when a particular feeling strikes you—pleasantly or unpleasantly. Notice and name what is happening right then and there and try to locate where in your body you feel it.

Feel Your Emotions Directly

You're already doing the preliminary work to feel your emotions directly. You're caring for your physical body by eating regularly and satisfyingly, prioritizing sleep, and beginning to understand your need for safety and connection. Perhaps you are meditating and feeling the breath with some consistency, which stabilizes the nervous system, slows things down, and helps you perceive signs of safety and danger more accurately.

These behaviors increase resilience and cognitive flexibility with which you can have real-time awareness. This allows you to interrupt the momentum of habitual reactions and instead respond in skillful and compassionate ways even when you are suffering. What follows are some practices to help you more naturally feel emotions directly.

1. Acknowledge Suffering

I love that Buddhist philosophy acknowledges suffering. I'm suspicious of toxic positivity and the near obsession with obliterating discomfort. Acknowledging suffering—rather than running from it, masking it, or trying to turn it into something else—is such a relief!

By acknowledging suffering, you have already stayed with it longer than you might have previously. I used to bolt as soon as I felt the slightest hint of discomfort. Most of the time, I never even registered I was uncomfortable because I so quickly ran from it. Acknowledging it, on the other hand, requires that you sit with it even if just for a moment.

Acknowledging suffering can be as simple as saying, "This is a moment of suffering." But please find words that feel trustworthy to you. Here are a few more ideas:

"This is so hard/painful/scary/unfamiliar to me."

"I am really struggling right now."

"I feel so uncomfortable right now."

"I really don't want to feel this way."

Acknowledging suffering can be like poking a hole in a big scary monster. You might notice less tension, more space, or some relief. Or not. But whatever you feel, it is true. And you are getting to know it.

2. Normalize Suffering

When you suffer, you probably feel isolated and alone. Feeling as if you are the only one struggling can add to the suffering of suffering.

Intellectually you know you aren't the only one who experiences painful emotions. But how can you know that for sure? How does it feel to acknowledge everyone struggles sometimes? In fact, many people are struggling with similar issues to you right now. Normalizing suffering can help this concept become embodied.

Stating "Everyone feels sad sometimes" or "Lots of people on the planet are grieving right now" or "Everyone has lost something or someone important during this pandemic" can remind you of this shared experience. You might even notice a subtle shift in bodily sensations: softening, spaciousness, gentleness.

If your suffering is specific to food, I feel the need to normalize this as well. I cannot tell you how many times I have heard some version of "I'm fifty years old, how pathetic is it I still can't figure out my food?!" It is not pathetic, silly, stupid, or any other denigrating word you might use. You did your best given the situation. And you are not alone. Not by a long shot. Many of the people you think have this figured out are actually struggling right now. So please, if this feels like you, offer yourself one of the following statements (or your own creation) whenever you feel isolated:

"I am not alone in my struggles with food and body, and I am now on a path to healing."

"Even though it can feel like this part of my life is broken beyond repair, there is always hope."

"I did my best with what I knew in the past; I'm still learning to relate to food and my body differently."

"Though I feel at times like I've lost my connection to Intuitive Eating, even that is part of my path."

3. Savor the Good

Before you dive into feeling "negative" emotions, it may be helpful to practice with ones that feel more pleasant. Savoring is a technique used in polyvagal theory to anchor into the nervous system's safe and connected ventral state. I think of it as marinating your brain in positive neurotransmitters and letting that goodness expand into your whole body.

When you feel a positive emotion, acknowledge its wonderfulness and drop into your body to savor the sensations. For example, when a spring breeze brushes along your back, feel the joy and note the response in your skin, brain, and heart. Taking the first sip of good coffee, feel your brain light up with pleasure, and notice the surge of pleasure in your chest. Stay with that for just a few moments at a time.

Celebrate what is gradually becoming more natural in your Intuitive Eating practice. I often begin sessions with "What is going well?" This practice helps you savor what you might otherwise gloss over as you focus on the next problem to be solved.

Another way to savor is to practice gratitude. A gratitude practice may involve noting things that you feel grateful for as you encounter them, or it may be a list you run through right before you go to sleep. I love how a gratitude practice expands your perspective to include the beautiful aspects of your life. In no way is it meant to erase whatever negative experiences you have. It reflects more accurately the full landscape—not all positive, not all negative. All very real and valuable.

4. Touch In with the Bad

When you regularly acknowledge and normalize suffering, and savor or express gratitude, you may wish to touch in with negative emotions. Touching uncomfortable emotions is not forcing yourself to suffer or self-flagellate. It is becoming familiar with an important part of your emotional experience, one you might have avoided for the most part in the past.

The exercises throughout this chapter provide ways to connect with those previously avoided emotions. Noticing and naming, recognizing your aversion to discomfort, feeling your emotions in the body—all of these help you touch the tenderness of painful emotions.

When you feel such emotions and want to self-medicate, you can choose to touch what is really going on. Use one of the previous exercises or simply sit with your hand on your heart, feeling your own warmth, and be there for yourself.

MINDFUL MOMENT: Cultivating Compassionate Self-Talk

How you speak to yourself is critical to developing, sustaining, and deepening your Intuitive Eating practice. The diet culture has taught you to adopt aggressive self-talk, the assumption being that pushing yourself is "motivating." When you speak to yourself this way—"What is *wrong* with you?" or "You're disgusting!"— rather than feeling motivated, you feel defeated. Never good enough. The underlying view linking self-aggression with motivation is that you are a problem to be fixed.

Cultivating compassionate instead of aggressive self-talk requires practice. By paying attention nonjudgmentally, you can hear when you automatically speak to yourself harshly. Recognizing this—like recognizing your attention has strayed from the feeling of the breath during meditation—you acknowledge it and redirect as needed, with gentleness and precision. In this case, that redirection can follow a specific formula:

1.   Acknowledge something has come up for you that feels difficult and provokes critical self-talk.

2.   Recognize the negative self-talk feels more natural because you have "practiced" it more.

3.   Recommit to gentleness, knowing it will become more natural over time.

4.   Reframe your response with kindness, recognition of the common experience of suffering, and mindfulness that neither adds nor takes away anything from the situation.

For example, if you pull on a pair of pants late in the pandemic and they don't close over your belly, you might notice yourself quickly spiraling into despair, perhaps saying something like, "Everyone else used this time to get fit, and look at you!!!" This is your cue to take a moment and a deep breath, recognize the discomfort that provoked a habitual response, recommit to self-compassion, and reframe with something like: "This feels so hard. The diet mentality has taught me this is exactly what I should avoid. This has been such a difficult year, and I'm certainly not the only one whose body has changed during the pandemic."

Amaya's Story

Amaya emailed me one evening after our session to say she was having a hard night. She had gotten into a conversation with her mom in which they discussed Amaya's anxiety and depression and how it related to her discomfort with her larger body. Amaya's mom, a lifetime and current dieter, suggested Amaya "just cut out the junk food," which was making her feel awful and probably not allowing her to lose weight. Amaya's question for me was whether she should follow her mom's advice. My response was: "I understand this is so hard. I think cutting out the foods that were triggers for you would only start the cycle over. My sense is you might be using these foods to self-medicate because you feel so alone in this process. Your mom is still dieting, your friends are all dieting. Only you have decided to break the cycle, but it's lonely and hard and confusing at times. The more you touch this sadness directly and allow yourself to feel it, the less effective food might become in alleviating your discomfort. You will eventually find your people as more become aware of Intuitive Eating, but this is a difficult time. You're doing everything right: working with me and your therapist, taking your meds, eating regularly and satisfyingly, prioritizing sleep and rest. You will get through this and come out the other side."

Understanding the biology of emotion empowers you to work directly with your emotions—to recognize what you feel any given moment and respond precisely, skillfully, and with kindness. Such a deep and nuanced practice continues to unfold for the rest of your life.

What Can You Celebrate?

- What did you learn about emotions and your biology?

- What connections can you already make regarding the physical sensations of emotion?

- How is noticing and naming becoming a part of your regular practice?

- What do you notice about how you are speaking to yourself?

CHAPTER 8

Tending to Emotional Hunger

In her book *Mindful Eating,* pediatrician and Zen Buddhist teacher Jan Chozen Bays writes about the different kinds of hunger. This includes heart hunger, the emotional hunger you feel when you have unmet needs, experience internal turmoil, and struggle with difficult feelings.

Tending to emotional hunger is not about getting you to eat less. Eating is a valid and sometimes effective way of self-soothing. But eating for emotional reasons should not be your only or main way to care for your tender heart. And eating when your true need is to express anger, to feel unconditionally accepted, or to be authentically seen and heard will never satisfy you.

Learning to detect and respond to emotional hunger is about meeting your *actual* need. There is a saying: "No amount of what you don't need will ever be enough." I think of this when working with clients who wonder why they continue to suffer, or magnify their suffering, when they self-medicate difficult emotions with food.

True self-care requires an ample supply of coping skills to settle, soothe, and tend to what dysregulates your nervous system. Mindfulness helps you develop self-literacy to consistently detect, interpret, and respond to your ever-changing needs. This increases confidence overall and in ways specific to your Intuitive Eating practice.

In the last chapter, you learned to work directly with your feelings. In this chapter, you'll learn to triage whenever your heart is signaling the need for attention:

1. Begin with the body: Are your basic needs being met?

2. Assess your emotions: Are your basic emotional needs being met?

3. Identify your acute need in this moment, whether related to or influenced by numbers one and two above or separate.

4. Cope through intentional and nonharmful distraction, mindful soothing, deepening personal exploration, and asking for help.

Let's examine each one in more detail.

1. Double-Check You're Getting the "Biological Basics"

Any time you experience emotional turmoil, review the biological basics. One constant is your need for adequate quality and quantity of sleep, proper hydration, and regular meals consisting of a balance of protein, carbohydrate, and fat. When biological needs aren't met consistently, your nervous system senses danger, which can elicit fear, anxiety, and other dysregulated feelings. The dysregulation that occurs when biological needs aren't met can easily be misinterpreted as emotional dysregulation—it *is* emotional to not have your physical needs met!

Review the following list to ensure your physical needs are being met:

- Am I getting about eight hours of sleep a night? Is the quality of my sleep good? Am I waking up during the night? Do I feel rested when I wake up?

- Am I drinking enough water? Am I using a lot of coffee, soda, or other sources of caffeine?

- Am I taking my medication as prescribed? Do I need to revisit dosage with my prescriber? Might seasonal, environmental, or life changes necessitate a change?

- Am I eating about every four hours? Am I getting too hungry sometimes?

- Am I getting a balance of protein, carbohydrate, and fat?

- Am I eating foods I like and find satisfying?

- Do I have an adequate variety of foods at home?

- Am I moving my body? Are any physical conditions such as pain or injury going unaddressed?

- Is there anything causing me to feel physically unsafe?

If one or more of your biological basics are lacking, please tend to them as best as you can. There may still be acute emotional needs, but stabilizing your body in these ways will help you have the resilience, cognitive flexibility, and compassion necessary to navigate them.

2. Assess Your Basic Emotional Needs

As an emotional being, your basic needs are not limited to your physical body. Community, connection, spirituality, intimacy, sensuality, touch, comfort, and pleasure are some of the things you need to feel human. If these needs are not regularly on your radar, you may be chronically deficient in basic emotional nourishment. Some questions to ask when you are feeling emotional distress include:

- Have I been in touch with friends and family?

- Have I been able to share with someone (friend, family member, therapist, etc.) what is really going on with me lately?

- What have I been doing for fun? What makes me laugh these days?

- Have I been doing the things that give me joy? Cooking, reading, dancing, painting, singing, learning something new, listening to music, or watching movies, for example.

- Other than food, where do I find pleasure and comfort?

- What am I doing these days that fills me with delight?

- Am I getting enough physical touch these days, whether through sexual relationships, other sensual touch, nonsexual touch, massage, self-massage, or masturbation?

- What am I doing for my spiritual self?

- What am I doing to connect with community, whether through AA, Al Anon, church, synagogue, meditation center, community center, volunteer work, affinity group, book club, or something else?

- What am I doing to manage my stress? Is my current stress level above or below average?

- How are my mindfulness and meditation practices going?

Even if you are not having a difficult time, these questions address the basic emotional needs all humans share. Check in with this list periodically to ensure you are meeting your needs for satisfying relationships, physical touch, pleasure, and community. When you have these things, by the way, getting through tough times feels a bit more manageable.

Phoebe's Story

Phoebe had recently decided not to pursue weight-loss surgery. She was well aware of the painful truth that people treated her better when she was in a smaller body but decided not to harm herself any further through anything the diet culture had to offer. Still, Phoebe struggled with her relationship with food, her cravings, the urge to binge, and accepting her body as it was. We emphasized the importance of staying with her discomfort to move through and transform it while meeting her basic needs.

Phoebe understood the contributors to her painful relationship with food—parents who "didn't get it," poor boundaries and disproportionate concern with taking care of others that led her to use food as self-care, inconsistent eating and stocking of food—and had a plan for how to work through these issues both logistically and emotionally. We emphasized regular meals and snacks, adequate sleep and water, and paying attention to stabilize her biologically so she was more capable of staying with herself during times of discomfort. On bad body image days, through difficult discussions with her parents, work stress, and run-ins with people from her dieting past, Phoebe continued to "get the basics" and to pay attention to what was arising in her body, heart, and mind.

3. Get Clear on Your True Need Right Now

What did you learn by first assessing your basic physical and emotional needs? Does this shed any light on how you are feeling right now? Is it possible your current experience, for example, is being influenced by a lack of sleep or feelings of isolation? Or are you meeting your physical and emotional needs and what you are experiencing now is separate from that?

In many cases, a combination of factors are at work. For example, you are struggling with body image, but when you take a step back you realize you are sleep deprived, about to get your period, and dealing with a lot of stress at work that is messing with your ability to eat regularly, leading to occasional binges. If this were the case, this is how we might approach it:

1. Address basic physical needs.

2. Acknowledge and attend to basic emotional needs.

3. Gently engage with your current acute emotional difficulties that are separate from numbers one and two above.

Following these steps might look like this:

1. Make an effort to get to bed slightly earlier and practice proper sleep hygiene by turning off screens an hour before bed, using aromatherapy like lavender to signal bedtime is approaching, taking a warm bath or shower to calm and soothe your nervous system, and doing a sleep meditation or some yoga to further relax your body and mind into sleep. Also, try to address whatever makes it difficult to prioritize sleep. If young children are climbing into bed at night, could you alternate with your partner to take them back to bed and settle them? If you regularly practice "revenge procrastination," in which you get your me time needs met when your body really needs

sleep, consider scheduling time on the weekend to catch up on movies or shows that interfere with rest when watched late on weeknights.

Track your period so you know when it is coming and recognize your specific pattern of physical and emotional symptoms. Connecting a physical or emotional experience to where you are in your cycle can be a huge relief. Emphasize sleep, eating regularly, and providing yourself with comfort and soothing during this time.

2. Talk to someone about the stress you are experiencing at work. Might you relieve your burden by lightening your workload, changing how you are working or who you are working with, and reality checking whether you're putting too much pressure on yourself? Give yourself permission to use convenient foods so you can eat regularly—heating up a frozen breakfast sandwich in the morning, packing apples and trail mix for snacks, protecting thirty minutes to eat lunch, scheduling a timer to remind you to break for snacks, pairing salad from a box with frozen pizza for dinner. Assess whether it's appropriate to add stress-relieving techniques such as yoga, meditation, or breathing exercises.

3. Begin with self-compassion to address your current body image struggles: acknowledge your suffering, normalize it based on what you know about how many people struggle with body image, and offer yourself kindness. Recognize how unmet physical and emotional needs can make this struggle feel even harder. Remind yourself of the nature of impermanence and that this specific feeling won't last. Consider whether it is time to directly address body image struggles with an Intuitive Eating practitioner, a community dedicated to Health at Every Size and Intuitive Eating, or a workbook focused on improving body image, such as Sonya Renee Taylor's *Your Body Is Not an Apology Workbook*.

All of the different parts of your experience are related. And this path brings your full experience into the light—it is valuable and you are worth the effort. By framing working with yourself in these ways, difficulties can start to feel manageable.

4. How Can You Mindfully Care for Yourself?

How to respond to emotional hunger includes nondestructive distraction, mindful soothing, personal exploration, and asking for help. This is not an exhaustive list; please consider it a starting point to meet your emotional needs with precision and gentleness.

Nondestructive Distraction

Nondestructive distraction is just what you might imagine: temporarily removing yourself from what you experience as painful without increasing your suffering. It can be absorbing, entertaining, or just different from what you don't want to focus on. In the Buddhist tradition, anything can be used in productive and nonproductive ways, so please use your good judgment to decide how and how much to distract yourself. Some of the soothing techniques discussed in the Mindful Soothing section that follows can also be distracting; the way they are discussed there is more mindful and present.

Games: Playing games on your phone, iPad, computer, or device like a Nintendo can pull you in and allow you to forget troubles for a little while. Decide whether a repetitive or challenging game feels more pleasing to you in the moment.

Movies: With so many genres, you have choices when distracting with a movie. I personally prefer horror movies, but many people love lighthearted or familiar films when they are struggling because they know what to expect.

TV Shows: There are endless options for TV series. One consideration when using TV to distract yourself is setting limits so binge-watching does not interfere with adequate quality and quantity of sleep.

Napping: One of my personal favorites, napping can be a nondestructive distraction that both allows time to pass when you are suffering and "fills the tank" if fatigue is exacerbating how you are perceiving the emotion.

MINDFUL MOMENT: Nondestructive Distractions Short List

In your journal, create a "short list" of nondestructive distractions to turn to in a pinch. Take a moment to quiet and connect with the body. Close your eyes lightly or keep them gently open. Consider a recent moment of emotional distress in which you needed a break. What games, movies, and TV shows might have been appealing at that time? What games, movies, and TV shows have you been meaning to check out that might serve as a nondestructive distraction when you need one? Notice their specific qualities. How can you ensure this distraction does not become destructive in any way? Write down the category, title, and any specific considerations in your journal and keep it handy.

Mindful Soothing

As you learned in chapter 2, your nervous system is constantly seeking safety. When in a dysregulated state of sympathetic or dorsal activation, certain practices can bring you back up to the regulated ventral state. Mindful soothing includes food. There will be times when using food to soothe is the right choice at the right moment. What is different about this approach from emotional overeating is the conscious choice to eat, the mindful attention paid while eating, and the freedom from guilt or shame.

Eating: Given the variety of emotions that are dysregulating, there are different considerations in soothing yourself with food. When I am feeling stressed, my favorite crunchy snack is Inca corn, that giant, tooth-breaking corn nut. Crunchy or chewy textures regulate the nervous system when it is in a fight-or-flight sympathetic state. If feeling lonely or unwell, on the other hand, you might wish to eat something creamy, warm, or soupy. Consider the specific foods, tastes, textures, temperatures, and densities that meet your specific emotional needs in different circumstances.

Music: There is an endless variety of music to soothe your nervous system, but different nervous systems find different types of music appealing. Consider what music you normally listen to. Is it similar to or different from the music you might opt for when feeling emotional turmoil? The answer might depend on the specific emotions you are feeling. Anger might awaken a desire for something loud and powerful, while sadness might create a longing for something slow and melodic.

Aromatherapy: Certain scents may be soothing to your nervous system. Lavender is the best-known aromatherapy used to calm body and mind. Other soothing scents include chamomile, bergamot, sage, lemon, rose, and ylang-ylang. By contrast, orange, lemon, peppermint, balsam fir, rosemary, and cinnamon may arouse the nervous system and feel energizing.

Movement: Whether you need to discharge fight-or-flight sympathetic energy or elevate collapsed dorsal energy, movement is a versatile tool. Ask yourself, *How do I want to feel in my body?* when considering using physical activity as a mindful soother. Refer to chapter 6 to review the different types of action that might be soothing to your nervous system when feeling difficult emotions.

Restorative yoga: Restorative yoga postures address imbalances affecting the mind-body. Restorative yoga is different from more vigorous forms of yoga. It is intentionally restful and allows the body to restore using specific postures and supports such as blankets and bolsters. This practice downregulates the sympathetic nervous system associated with states of fight or flight and upregulates the parts of the nervous system connected with rest, calm, and rejuvenation.

Sensuality: Whether your emotion is directly related to a need for sensuality or not, engaging in consensual, fulfilling sex, masturbation, or massage can be extremely soothing for the nervous system. This is a topic often left out of resources such as this one, but we are essentially sexual and sensual beings. So please do what you can to consider this in a way that feels safe and authentic.

Breathing exercises: Clearly the breath is a powerful way of connecting mind and body. It is also an immediate way to soothe the nervous system. The breath is directly related to heart rate, with a slight speeding up during the inhale and a slight slowing down during the exhale. Elongating your exhale—breathing in for a count of four and out for a count of eight, for example—can communicate safety to your body. For other breath work techniques, seek out the support of a trained teacher.

Compression: Deep pressure therapy such as firm hugging, firm stroking, squeezing, or swaddling can calm a dysregulated nervous system. The most popular form of compression used these days is a weighted blanket, which should weigh about 10 percent of your body weight. Compression may help relieve anxiety and improve sleep.

Body care: It can feel dismissive when you are suffering and someone tells you to take a warm bath. But when a warm bath or shower, a manicure and pedicure, or splashing cold water on your face is exactly what your body is asking for, it can be very regulating.

Other sensory stimulation: Tending to the senses in other ways not named above may be regulating to you. Putting on the softest and most comfortable clothing you possess, intentionally touching specific textures such as faux fur or the softest silk, lying on an acupressure mat, or squeezing a stress ball are all valid tools to add to your mindful soothing toolbox. You can come up with more of your own as you continue to deepen your attunement to your needs.

MINDFUL MOMENT: What Are Your Go-to Mindful Soothing Techniques?

In your journal, identify at least three soothing techniques that are appealing. Come to a quiet seated position and connect with your body. Consider a time when you were struggling emotionally and imagine what mindful soothing technique might have been supportive to you. Would you opt for food or music or some form of sensory stimulation? Would you try a weighted blanket or putting on sneakers and walking out the door? Would you splash cold water on your face or take a warm bath? What specific attributes appeal to you and why? Don't wait for a distressing emotion to come along to use these techniques. Experiment with them right away so you can start to collect data on what helps and what doesn't. Create a list of techniques in your journal and update the list as you conduct your experiments.

Personal Exploration

Noticeably different from distracting and soothing, personal exploration involves moving toward your discomfort in accessible ways. You might choose behaviors from this list when you feel safe and stable enough to directly engage with what is happening in your life but perhaps not yet ready to ask for help. Many of the options normalize what you are experiencing, which may allow shame to dissipate so that you can reach out to others for support.

Reading: Books, articles, and specific Intuitive Eating–aligned social media accounts may provide supportive content that both addresses your in-the-moment feelings and provides ideas about a way forward. A list of suggested resources is provided at http://www.newharbinger.com/49401.

Self-help books are not the only options here (and clearly I have no objection to self-help books!). Memoir, fiction, and nonfiction social commentary can also create incredible connections and feelings of being seen and understood.

Listening/participating: Podcasts, webinars, and platforms like Clubhouse let you listen to experts discuss their subjects. You may also hear the personal experiences of others dealing with similar feelings. The pandemic engendered an incredible number of remote classes. When focused on letting go of dieting, living an anti-diet life, and improving body image, these courses offer not only specific guidance and reflection but also community and connection with others. A partial list of suggested podcasts and courses is provided at http://www.newharbinger.com/49401.

Journaling: Many writers write to figure out how they feel; they don't come to the page knowing exactly what they are going to write. Similarly, writing may allow you to discover what is going on inside. There are various approaches to journaling, including unstructured writing, responding to prompts, and morning pages.

Unstructured writing could be done at regular times each day or irregularly when the mood strikes. There is no guidance on what to write. Journaling prompts, on the other hand, suggest a topic or contemplation to stimulate your writing. Consider the topics listed under Contemplations below for some ideas. Morning pages are a practice introduced by Julia Cameron in her book *The Artist's Way*. Morning pages consists of writing three pages longhand every morning to dump out whatever arises from the mind to the page. It is often done as part of a morning routine that may include a meditation and creative writing practice.

Workbooks: Workbooks provide a framework to approach topics such as self-compassion or acceptance and commitment therapy. They can be done in a structured or unstructured way, whether you complete them sequentially, jump around, or only access them when you feel the need. The beauty of workbooks is they help you take concepts into embodied practice. Some of my favorites include:

- *The Intuitive Eating Workbook* (4th edition) by Evelyn Tribole and Elyse Resch, 2017

- *The Mindful Self-Compassion Workbook* by Kristin Neff and Christopher Germer, 2018

- *ACT Made Simple: An Easy-to-Read Primer on Acceptance and Commitment Therapy* by Russ Harris and Steven C. Hayes, 2019

- *Your Body Is Not an Apology Workbook: Tools for Radical Self-Love* by Sonya Renee Taylor, 2021

Meditations: Substituting for your discursive mind another object of attention is a definition of meditation I hold dear. The following is a list of different ways to focus your attention. Instructions can be found at http://www.newharbinger.com/49401.

- Shamatha: an open-eye breath awareness practice of feeling, allowing, and being with yourself. Instructions can be found in chapter 1.

- Lovingkindness: a meditation in which you wish for safety, health, happiness, and a life of ease for yourself, a loved one, a neutral person, an enemy, and ultimately all beings.

- Compassion: a meditation in which you offer wishes for the relief of suffering for yourself, a loved one, a neutral person, an enemy, and ultimately all beings.

- Self-compassion: a variety of practices in which you offer kindness to yourself.

- Tonglen: also known as the practice of sending and taking, this meditation guides you to breathe in suffering and breath out relief.

- Gratitude: a practice in which you intentionally appreciate what you are grateful for.

Contemplations: In contemplations, you place your attention on a specific statement or idea. When the mind wanders, you bring your attention back to that object. When you do contemplations, begin and end with five minutes or so of shamatha meditation to settle the body and mind. Some ideas to contemplate include:

- "My body is okay as it is."

- "I am the only expert of my body."

- "I am one of millions challenging the diet culture."

- "I can be with difficult emotions."

- "It matters that I am feeling, allowing, and being with my strong emotions."

- "The world is moving toward Intuitive Eating."

In your journal, identify two forms of personal exploration that appeal to you. Come to a quiet seated position and connect with your body. Consider something you are currently working with and imagine how you might explore it. Does journaling appeal to you? What kind? Could you imagine delving into a workbook or exploring a concept in a contemplation? Don't wait for whatever issue you are working with to become a crisis. Try engaging with it through personal exploration now and see how that affects the trajectory of your experience.

Asking for Help

Asking for help may look different at different times. Who and how you ask for help has everything to do with your specific needs at the time. Consider the list below as a starting point because going into adequate detail is beyond the scope of this book. Contemplate your needs or discuss them with someone you trust to determine what steps you can take to care for your tender heart.

Relationships: Sometimes the people you need support from are right there in front of you. Your spouse, roommate, friend, parent, sibling—the people you interact with most may be the ones to make a difference as you embark on or deepen an Intuitive Eating practice and tend to the deeper emotional wounds you've suffered. Setting boundaries, teaching others how to support you, helping them understand what is not supportive—these are difficult conversations to have. Due to the closeness and importance of these individuals, staying with that discomfort and expressing your needs authentically can have a positive ripple effect in your life.

Therapy: Talking to a trained expert, processing and reframing your experiences, and finding new ways of thinking and behaving in your life are all elements of therapy. The following is a non-exhaustive list of some forms of therapy particularly relevant to issues around food and body:

- Accelerated experiential dynamic psychotherapy (AEDP): A technique in which the client and therapist cocreate a present, healing relationship emphasizing real-time body-based processing of difficult emotions.

- Acceptance and commitment therapy (ACT): A form of psychotherapy in which you accept circumstances, process your responses, and commit to taking actions aligned with your deepest values.

- Cognitive behavioral therapy (CBT): A psychosocial intervention focusing on reframing thoughts so you can make positive behavioral changes.

- Dialectical behavior therapy (DBT): Derived from CBT, DBT incorporates distress tolerance, emotional regulation, and mindfulness techniques to create positive behavioral change.

- Emotionally focused therapy (EFT): A form of therapy focusing on adult relationship patterns and attachment to establish trust and move relationships in a positive direction.

- Family systems therapy: A form of therapy that addresses dynamics in the family unit to identify and resolve personal and relationship challenges.

- Internal family systems therapy (IFS): A form of psychotherapy in which each individual comprises "parts," many of which have been wounded, that serve different functions to create harmony and healing for the whole person.

- Mindfulness-based cognitive therapy: A derivative of CBT using mindfulness and meditation to reframe negative thoughts and promote positive change.

- Motivational interviewing (MI): A counseling method acknowledging the difficulty of and ambivalence toward change that harnesses an individual's internal motivation for change.

- Somatic therapy: A body-based therapy combining talking, mind-body exercises, and physical techniques such as deep breathing to relieve symptoms associated with trauma.

Medication: Antidepressants, antianxiety meds, mood stabilizers, medications to help you sleep, medications to calm the nervous system while you work through your trauma—there are many options to consider based on your specific needs. There can still be stigma around taking medication for anything related to mental health, but these perspectives are based in ignorance and fear. If you think you might benefit from medication for depression, anxiety, or any other form of mental illness, speak with your internist, primary care physician, or (ideally) a psychiatrist. People often experience some symptom relief after making the decision to take a medication. You might discover that medication allows you to do the deeper emotional work that felt inaccessible beforehand.

Alternative therapies: Alternative therapies have come a long way from dietary supplements and yoga. If you feel you have already tried everything and are still struggling, please know there are still many options worth exploring. From off-label uses of medications, experimental therapies, and nonpharmacologic approaches such as transcranial magnetic stimulation, the world of modalities providing options in mental health continues to grow. Speak to a professional, such as a psychiatrist (whom I've always found to be the most knowledgeable about alternative therapies), about what might be right for you.

There is no need to get to a point of deeper suffering to engage help from others. How can you increase your sources of support now and develop a contingency plan for how you could ask for support at a later time?

MINDFUL MOMENT: Mindfully Asking for Help

Come to a quiet seated position and connect with your body. Consider where you are on your Intuitive Eating and mindfulness journey. In your journal, respond to the following prompts:

- How could I imagine eventually asking for help?

- Where are the gaps in my support system?

- What is missing from my self-care arsenal: medication, therapy, conversations with family and friends about how to specifically support me?

Tending to your emotional needs—your heart hunger—takes your Intuitive Eating practice to a much deeper level. It is often the bridge between the practice that just affects your relationship with food and body and the practice that impacts the rest of your life. Discerning when your hunger is physical and when it is emotional—and knowing in a deep and embodied way what you truly need—only fortifies your trust in your own body, mind, and heart. And it prepares you to finally make lasting peace with food.

What Can You Celebrate?

- In what ways are you already tending to your emotional hunger?

- How would you like to care for yourself emotionally?

- What methods of distracting, soothing, exploring, and asking for help feel accessible now?

- What methods of distracting, soothing, exploring, and asking for help might become appealing in the future?

CHAPTER 9

Finding Peace with Food

Finding peace with food is possible with Intuitive Eating and mindfulness! Read that one again.

Your body's natural capacity for self-regulation is synonymous with this peace. When you relate to food from an uncomplicated place, you recognize food as just food—each with a slightly different combination of protein, carbohydrate, and fat. A variety of tastes, temperatures, and textural components. No inherent moral superiority or inferiority to any other food. A source of pleasure and sustenance. Sometimes spectacular, sometimes meh.

How you seek peace with food is as important as the actual peace. There is a big difference between doing this work as self-improvement and doing it as self-care. A self-improvement approach to peace with food implies you must get rid of the noise and charge around food because it can lead to weight gain. Making peace as a means of self-care suggests you are worth facing the discomfort and worth the effort of staying with yourself through every part of your experience.

The war with food comes in many varieties and the peace process must take all of them into account:

- The discomfiting tension of believing certain foods are dangerous and can make you gain weight and get sick

- The cognitive dissonance of getting signals from your body that conflict with messages from the diet culture

- The dread of the gravitational pull toward a binge when you are chronically undereating

- The belief that once you start eating, you'll never stop

- The shame of eating your feelings and not knowing other ways to soothe yourself

- The humiliation of feeling food is your only friend, your only indulgence, your only source of comfort and pleasure

The antidotes to the war with food, the ways to find lasting and genuine peace, begin with everything you've learned so far:

- Feeding yourself regularly, adequately, and satisfyingly

- Giving yourself continuous unconditional permission to eat

- Sensing, interpreting, and tending to your emotional needs

- Speaking to yourself with tenderness and compassion

- Reminding yourself that this path is all process

In this chapter, you'll learn how mindfulness can take these already familiar practices deeper. Be prepared to connect the dots between thoughts, feelings, and actions to understand your experience and move toward more authentic self-care. You'll also practice making peace with specific charged foods and quantities of foods.

Peace of any kind comes when you feel safe. Before diving into this chapter, address whether or not you feel safe and secure enough to do so at this time.

MINDFUL MOMENT: Safety Check

In this practice, you will be stilling the body to assess whether your overall perception is one of safety or danger. Take a few moments to come to a comfortable seated or lying down position. Let your eyes rest open or gently closed. Take a few embodied breaths, focusing your mind's attention on the feeling of breath coming into and going out of the body.

Scanning the body slowly from the bottom of your feet up to the crown of your head, notice any sensations. Notice any sensations associated with danger: restlessness, agitation, tension, disconnection, numbness, feelings of vulnerability, fear, or a sinking feeling. Notice any sensations associated with safety: grounded-ness, centeredness, stillness, calm, warmth, relaxation, or a settled or comfort-able feeling.

To the sensations and parts of your body feeling unsafe, offer compassion and gentleness. Thank your nervous system for protecting you. Reassure your body you will protect it in return. Close this practice with a few minutes of sha-matha meditation, feeling the breath, allowing the mind to be as it is, redirecting your attention when it gets lost.

If now is the time to pursue peace with food, review the following list to ensure this is a reasonable thing to ask of yourself at this time given what else is going on in your life. It can also help you identify the source(s) of your internal war. Return to this list any time your sense of peace with food feels threatened.

Are You Feeding Yourself Regularly, Adequately, and Satisfyingly?

When you're consistently fed—regularly and adequately, to the point of fullness and satisfaction—food and eating become less emotionally charged and more straightforward. When you are not, your body senses danger and your thinking can become distorted.

Eating regularly means, for the most part, you are not veering into the danger zone of extreme hunger where eating and thinking speed up and become chaotic. Eating adequately includes finding a balance of protein, carbohydrate, and fat and reaching a point of comfortable fullness that feels like enough to you. Eating satisfyingly implies you are eating the foods you want to eat and that you find pleasurable, meeting your unique needs for taste, temperature, texture, density, and filling capacity. Consider whether any of the following factors are making it difficult to eat regularly, adequately, and satisfyingly and potentially contributing to the war with food:

- Examples of obstacles to eating regularly:

  - Scheduling problems such as inflexible work expectations

  - Raising young kids without adequate support

  - Inconsistent schedule that makes it difficult to find a routine

  - Difficulty keeping track of time

  - Difficulty connecting with sensations of hunger

  - Inadequate stock of foods at home

  - Difficulty accessing food away from home

  - Food insecurity

- Examples of obstacles to eating adequately:

  - Residual diet mentality telling you less is more

  - Feeling surveilled by people you eat with

  - Feeling you have to compete with others for food

  - Comparing with others how much you need to eat to feel full

  - Food insecurity

- Examples of obstacles to eating satisfyingly:

  - Inadequate stock of foods

  - Inadequate variety of foods available

  - Internal or external judgments about food choices

  - Residual diet mentality telling you certain foods are bad or off-limits

  - Difficulty imagining which foods might contribute to satisfaction

  - Limited experience with a variety of foods

  - Food insecurity

Food insecurity exists on all three lists for good reason: if you do not have secure and consistent access to a variety of foods, it is not reasonable to try to make peace with food right now. Food insecurity is a traumatic and very common experience that alters your ability to feel safe, let alone your ability to transform diet mentality. If this describes your experience, consider accessing resources for food insecurity and support for trauma. Food banks, food pantries, food drives, community centers, community gardens, community fridges, social service agencies, and houses of worship are just a few.

Assessing whether you are feeding yourself regularly, adequately, and satisfyingly provides valuable information about how to make peace with food. If you aren't eating regularly, implement a structured eating approach as described in chapter 3 for a couple of weeks and note any changes before coming back to this chapter. If you are not consistently eating adequately, go back to chapter 4 to refamiliarize yourself with what level of fullness feels like "enough" and how to address barriers to respecting that. If you are not satisfied with your eating experiences, review chapter 5 to introduce the tastes, textures, temperatures, and sustaining capacities that contribute to true satisfaction, ensuring you regularly have access to such a variety.

MINDFUL MOMENT: Prioritizing Your Preferences

Grab your journal. Think of three foods you enjoy. These don't have to be your absolute favorites or foods that are particularly charged for you (unless you want to explore those). Consider what makes these foods particularly enjoyable for you. What are the tastes, textures, temperatures, densities, eating environments, and other qualities that make eating enjoyable? Get as specific as possible.

For example, if cornbread is one of your foods, I'd ask you:

- Do you prefer it sweet, savory, or neutral?

- What size crumb do you like? Very fine or more granular?

- How dry versus moist do you like it?

- Do you like other "stuff" in your cornbread, like jalapeños?

- What thickness do you prefer?

- Do you like it in muffins or cut from a larger piece?

- Do you like to eat it alone or alongside other foods?

This might seem like a lot of detailed questions, but it's important to prioritize your specific idiosyncratic tastes. To acknowledge they matter. This is not being picky. It's yet another form of self-care that values your body's innate intelligence.

Rebecca's Story

Rebecca usually fasted on Yom Kippur but then inevitably binged when she broke the fast. The public nature of her binges were particularly shame-inducing. After reading a social media post by a Jewish woman in recovery, Rebecca decided to experiment with not fasting during the holiday. As she thought through this experiment, we addressed what might come up:

> *How would she observe the holiday?* Express her atonement by contemplating and journaling about the ways in which she might have harmed others, including herself through dieting.

> *How would she explain her decision?* Describe how she had given the matter great consideration and decided she could observe the holiday more authentically if she was not starving herself.

> *How would she eat when she broke the fast?* As she would eat at any meal—finding an enjoyable balance of tastes and textures, especially the foods unique to the holiday.

Rebecca challenged old ways of thinking to prioritize eating regularly, adequately, and satisfyingly. As the result of her experiment, she found she was much more able to focus on the true meaning of the holiday. Rebecca also really enjoyed the meal afterward without feeling like she overdid it.

Are You Continually Reinforcing Unconditional Permission to Eat?

Dieting messages have been coursing through your neurons for years, maybe decades. It takes time and practice to change them. Giving yourself unconditional permission to eat does not happen all at once. You must reinforce this permission again and again, during individual eating experiences and overall in a larger sense. When the time feels right to make peace with food, assess whether you have truly given yourself unconditional permission to eat, whether you have lapses or exceptions, and whether you are practicing some form of what Evelyn Tribole and Elyse Resch call "pseudodieting."

Unconditional permission to eat is not eating whatever you want, whenever you want, and in any amount you want. And it is not overwhelming your taste buds with a particular food so you eventually grow sick of it. Dieting doesn't meet your personal and ever-changing needs, and neither would doing the opposite and giving no thought to what, when, and how much you eat. Unconditional permission to eat is a middle way in which you truly believe—body and mind—that no food is off-limits or better than another food and you deserve to eat what you really want when you want it. Then you can finally figure out what satisfies you.

Ask yourself these questions to determine whether you are giving yourself full and unconditional permission to eat:

- Are there certain foods you can't stop eating once you begin? Are there foods you fear will affect you in this way?

- Are there foods you restrict in some way because you don't trust yourself around them, whether by not buying them or keeping them around, giving away food gifts, or avoiding places that sell them?

- Are there certain foods you claim not to like when the truth is more complicated?

- Are there certain foods you claim will make you sick when the truth is more complicated?

- Are there certain foods you believe are not appropriate to eat if you are in a larger body?

- Are there certain foods you eat differently depending on who you're with?

- Are there foods that provoke guilt or remorse when you eat them?

- Are there foods you cannot eat without questioning whether you should?

- Are there certain foods you limit quantities of rather than allowing your body to determine how much feels like enough?

- Do you regularly predetermine how much you will eat during an eating experience rather than allowing your body to determine how much you need to eat to feel satisfied?

- Are there certain meals or settings at which you consistently eat past fullness?

If you answer yes to one or more, making peace with food likely involves reinforcing your unconditional permission to eat. Mindful exposure therapy in which you intentionally and systematically habituate to charged foods and experiment with comfortable fullness can help.

MINDFUL MOMENT: Mindfully Making Peace with Charged Foods

Get your journal. Identify the foods you thought of for the questions above. Rank them in order of charge, with the least charged foods at the bottom and the most charged at the top.

Choose one of the foods from your list, beginning with something in the moderate range. Identify the specific brand and flavor and prioritize the version of the food you most enjoy. Do not vary the flavor or brand so you can focus your attention on this one version and observe any changes in your experience of eating it.

Determine how you will eat the food:

- Find a time when you are not too hungry, perhaps a 2 on your hunger scale.

- Find a time when your stress level is not elevated, you've gotten enough sleep, and you've been eating regularly.

- Decide whether you want support from anyone and have that discussion or find time when you can be alone.

- Determine where you will obtain the food. If it is something you will be eating at home, make sure you have plenty of the food stocked. For example, if you chose Ben and Jerry's Chubby Hubby ice cream, have three pints in your freezer at all times. If you finish one, get another to replace it.

When you're ready, find a peaceful place with no distractions. Take a few moments to settle your body, taking three deep embodied breaths and feeling the sensations of each inhale and exhale. Notice any sensations in your body as you prepare to eat the food. Is there excitement, fear, anticipation? Record what you notice.

As you eat the food, stay connected with your physical senses. Whenever you get lost in thoughts about eating the food—any narratives or judgments—use the shamatha technique to gently guide your attention back to your present-moment body. Record in your journal what you notice about the taste, texture, and other sensory characteristics of the food. Is it what you hoped for? Better? Worse? How does the eating experience change even subtly with each bite?

After eating the food, notice any sensations. Do you feel fullness and/or satisfaction? Can you be curious and nonjudgmental? If you notice judgments or stories, note them as well and identify them as such. Repeat this exercise as many times as necessary to begin to notice a shift. Give this adequate time to happen; it may be a month or more. Lean on your meditation practice to help stabilize and support your capacity for presence and awareness.

MINDFUL MOMENT: Mindfully Making Peace with Comfortable Fullness

Get that journal again. If you regularly eat beyond comfortable fullness, identify the circumstances in which this happens:

- At breakfast, lunch, snacks, or dinner? During the food preparation stage such as before dinner or between meals?

- When you are alone or with others?

- Are there certain foods associated with your eating beyond comfortable fullness?

- Are there certain settings at which this is more likely to happen, for example, at restaurants, at your parents' house, at Friday night dinners, after Sunday service, etc.?

Once you understand the circumstances in which you eat beyond comfortable fullness, identify one scenario to experiment with. Do this on a day you have the greatest chance of mindfulness: you have slept well, you've been eating regularly, and your stress level is average or below.

As you approach the meal or situation, come into your body and assess what you are feeling. Find a comfortable seated position and lightly close your eyes or leave them gently open. Take three deep breaths, focusing your mind's attention on the sensation of the breath coming in and going out through the nose. What sensations do you notice? Are you amped up, feeling restless, with energy coursing through your body? Are you feeling low and slow and in need of a pick-me-up? Record "noticings" in your journal.

As you eat, focus attention on the sensory aspects of the food, noticing subtle changes bite to bite. Are you enjoying the food? Check in with hunger and fullness every few minutes and note changes.

When you get to a place that feels like comfortable fullness, take another moment to check in. Take another intentional breath and focus on that sensation. What do you feel in your body overall, your stomach, your mouth? What is the level of desire to keep eating? How does the food taste and has that changed? Do you feel ready to experiment with stopping now?

If not, please do not despair. You will get there by repeating this experiment. If you do feel ready, sit back in your chair and rest with that decision. Notice emotions and sensations that arise in your body. Notice sadness, disappointment, or resistance. Whatever you feel is normal. Can you sit with it without judgment?

You always have permission to eat. If, after a break, you wish to eat more, sit with that desire before acting on it. What is that like? If you decide not to continue to eat, what thoughts, emotions, and sensations arise?

You can also notice micromoments of peace with food throughout your day in an unstructured way. When you have an enjoyable bite of food, a taste or texture exactly hits the spot, or something you're eating is not exactly as you like, this is a moment of peaceful awareness to appreciate.

Are You Sensing, Interpreting, and Tending to Emotional Needs?

Making peace with food requires tending to physical and emotional needs regularly, precisely, and as they occur. Because many people struggle to work directly with their emotions, those needs gets tangled up with eating in a distressing way.

Many people use food to manage difficult emotions. There is nothing wrong with seeking comfort from food. Food is definitely comforting and can be one tool in soothing a dysregulated nervous system. But if eating is the only way of responding to difficult feelings, imagine all the emotional needs that go unmet.

Here is a classic way in which eating and emotions collide:

1. A difficult emotion arises, such as anger, sadness, grief, or general ickiness.

2. You suddenly desire something crunchy, sweet, salty, creamy, a forbidden food, or leftovers.

3. You eat but not in an enjoyable way because the eating is rapid, pressured, and desperate.

4. You feel shame, guilt, and remorse about eating or you feel physically and emotionally numb.

Remember how I keep saying your nervous system exists to protect you? Well, this is another example. Eating in response to strong dysregulating emotions is an attempt to regulate. Strong emotions may feel dangerous; eating can discharge sympathetic energy or elevate collapsed dorsal energy. When you don't know what else to do, this is a smart way to feel safe. Please have compassion for that part of you trying to feel safe.

Many people gravitate toward "sugar" when feeling strong emotions and my response is always the same: we don't come out of the womb knowing how to self-regulate; we need our adults to co-regulate for us. But we do come out of the womb liking sweet things, so good for you for figuring out you can feel safe and good by eating something sweet.

Nicole's Story

Nicole was diagnosed with type 1 diabetes when she was nine. The trauma of that diagnosis and how it meant a completely different lifestyle for her than any of her peers was never explicitly addressed with family, doctors, teachers, or anyone. Without support to process, Nicole put the pieces together as best as she could with a nine-year-old brain: her body was defective, sugar was dangerous, everyone else could safely have sugar but her.

That narrative persisted into adulthood. She was both afraid of sugar and drawn to it, bingeing when she felt stressed or anxious. If she experienced high or low blood sugar, Nicole felt guilt and shame, as if she should be able to prevent any fluctuation. We worked together to destigmatize sugar so she could enjoy it in a way that didn't dramatically affect her blood sugar and to develop a variety of coping strategies other than eating. By eating high-sugar foods along with sources of protein, fat, and fiber, Nicole could enjoy the foods she feared. By compiling a list of coping skills—listening to podcasts, meditating, practicing self-compassion, using a weighted blanket—she had options other than self-soothing with food.

Refer to the coping skills outlined in chapter 8 for ideas on tending directly to emotional needs so they don't get distorted and tangled up with eating behaviors. Whether you need nondestructive distraction, mindful soothing, personal exploration, or support from someone else, you will be accumulating life skills.

You might also try some of the following techniques to regulate quickly:

- Chanting, such as sounding the "Voo" syllable at the bottom of your vocal range, to produce a vibration in your neck and chest

- Singing or humming

- Gargling with warm water

- Splashing cold water on your face, taking a cold shower, going outside for a walk in the cold

- Slowing and deepening your breath for five to ten minutes with an emphasis on lengthening the exhale

- Facial massage, foot massage, full-body massage

- Meditating

- Laughing

- Being around another nervous system that feels safe (ideally someone with whom you experience delight)

Are You Speaking to Yourself with Tenderness and Compassion?

As you pursue peace with food, self-talk matters. With patience and practice, a shift will take place. For example, when you try something new and it doesn't work out as you hoped, you might initially and automatically speak to yourself harshly, but even this is an opportunity to course-correct.

Consider this example: You decide to experiment with making peace with your favorite kind of candy—Reese's Peanut Butter Cups. You get a couple of bags so there's no risk of running out. The first time, it's after a satisfying lunch so you are at the perfect hunger level to experiment with this charged food. You follow all my guidance for checking in with yourself physically and emotionally, you eat without distraction, but after the first two, things speed up rather than slow down. You eat eight of them and feel uncomfortable and frustrated. Now you have some options.

Option A might sound most familiar. When an eating experience ends in physical discomfort and frustration, your go-to self-talk sounds like this: "What is wrong with you? You can't stop after two of them, which is the serving size and the amount you *should* have been satisfied with. You have no self-control and that will never change. You might as well eat the rest of them and go back to your original strategy of never keeping them in the house."

Option B will sound unfamiliar at first: "That was not what you expected. You were hoping the first time you tried this, you would immediately feel satisfied with less but that's not what happened. This makes sense: you've deprived yourself for a long time and you are still in the process of convincing your body and your mind that these are not off-limits. Each time you do this experiment, that will get a little clearer. For now, give yourself credit for trying, for having hope, for confronting your fear directly. This is exactly how you change. You are doing everything right."

Option B is how I would speak to you. You might even imagine me there with you saying these words at first. With time, the voice will sound like your own.

Even if you begin with Option A, you can respond to that with compassion. You can have compassion for the part of you that struggles to have compassion for yourself! Self-aggressive statements might come first for a while, and that's okay. How you respond to them matters.

MINDFUL MOMENT: Reframing Self-Talk

Journal time. Think of an aggressive or critical statement you repeat to yourself. Write it down. Read it back to yourself. Say it out loud. How does that feel in your body and heart to hear those words?

Imagine I'm sitting there with you. What would I say? How would I say it? Write down those words. Read them back to yourself. Say them out loud. How do your body and heart feel? Can you trust these words? What could make them more trustworthy?

Each time you hear self-aggressive or critical statements, come back to this exercise. How could you reframe them in a way that is both compassionate and trustworthy?

Are You Remembering That This Path Is All Process?

You've probably heard the saying, "Life is a journey, not a destination." This strikes me as particularly Buddhist and essential to Intuitive Eating, with emphasis on being where you are, not on outcome.

You probably came to this work with an outcome in mind. You want to stop thinking about food so much or to feel more confident in your choices. Focusing on a particular outcome is actually an obstacle. Projecting into the future—about how you will think or act or feel around and about food—instantly takes you out of the moment.

This is why focus on weight loss is inherently in conflict with mindfulness. Even the emphasis on "figuring out your food" can obstruct present-moment awareness that might lead you to figure out your food. It's not a problem to wish for specific outcomes. When you do, notice yourself fast-forwarding into the future, and bring yourself back to determine what you are feeling right then and there and what you need.

You are already an Intuitive Eater. You are already having Intuitive Eating experiences every day. These don't have to be earth-shattering realizations. Better they be small and cumulative.

MINDFUL MOMENT: Inventory of Past Challenges and Celebrations

Another journal moment for you. You will be compiling a list of past challenges you have attended to and resolved to some degree. Do this exercise when struggling with something specific or generally questioning your capacity for peace with food. Review this compilation of your Intuitive Eating celebrations (the subtler, the better) when you just need a boost.

Some examples:

- When you struggle to identify what you are hungry for, recall any moments in which you chose something that exactly "hit the spot."

- When you struggle to feel safe around certain charged foods, recall the foods with which you struggled in the past and have made peace.

- If you binge, recall moments you intentionally fed yourself regularly or even moments during the binge when you were present.

By revisiting past accomplishments over time, you realize progress has been happening all along, often when you're not aware of it.

What Can You Celebrate?

- How are you increasing your chances for peace with food?

- What are some subtle moments of Intuitive Eating to recall when you are struggling?

- How are you transforming and reframing self-talk?

PART III

Mindfulness of Mind

With mindfulness of mind, you *identify* your thoughts about food, eating, your body, and weight and then you *de-identify with* them. You are not your thoughts! They do not define who you are or what you do.

Mindfulness lets you observe the relationship between beliefs, thoughts, feelings, and behaviors, and redirect toward gentleness, compassion, and kindness. Toward being with yourself and your experiences as they are.

Acknowledging thoughts as "just thought," releasing them gently and precisely, and coming back to your present-moment experience invites spaciousness, permission, forgiveness, and wisdom to arise.

CHAPTER 10

How Mindfulness Affects Your Thoughts

Many of us feel identified with and attached to our thoughts as if they were *the truth.* "We think, therefore we are," to riff on the famous Descartes quote. This attachment means temporary thoughts sweeping through our minds determine *who we think we are, how we feel,* and *what we do.* This feels particularly true within the diet mentality.

Casey's Story

Casey had been practicing Intuitive Eating for several months. Eating according to hunger, recognizing emerging fullness, moving in ways that were fun and invigorating, and prioritizing satisfaction were becoming natural practices for her. She continued to want to lose weight and felt shame about this. One day, in preparation for an in-person meeting, Casey stepped on the scale to see whether her weight had changed with Intuitive Eating. She discovered she had lost a few pounds and immediately felt better.

At the meeting, Casey felt confident and outgoing. She realized how much she missed being in a room with real people. When colleagues shared pictures from the event, Casey was crestfallen because she didn't like how she looked. Rather than going down a shame spiral, Casey took this opportunity to observe how quickly thoughts could change based on outside influences. This helped Casey reinforce her allegiance to her internal perspective and her intelligent body.

Because the diet culture is "the water you swim in," you internalize its system of thought. Even though the commonly held definition of beauty has changed over the last several centuries—suggesting there is no objective meaning of beauty—you probably identify with the current one. It makes sense; this is all you have known. In your mind, thinness equals beauty, health, desirability, and happiness. Had you lived a hundred years ago, your thoughts would be different. One hundred years from now, they would be different as well.

In the Buddhist tradition, your thoughts are separate from who you are. Your mind is described as the blue sky, constant and unchanging, while thoughts are the temporary clouds passing by. Clouds can be light and fluffy one day and dark and threatening another. Sometimes the clouds might completely obscure the sky, but it is still there, unchanged. Other times the sky is uncharacteristically clear. This is the nature of mind. So don't believe everything you think!

Meditation Changes Your Relationship to Thought

Mindfulness in general, and meditation in particular, makes working with thought possible, no matter how distressing. It provides the model for how to work with diet mentality thoughts in all their sneaky iterations. One analogy for meditation is sitting in a train station watching the trains (of thought) go by. The practice is to sit and observe but not get on any of the trains. If at some point you realize you did get on a train, get off as soon as you can and resume watching.

The meditation technique you learned in chapter 1 transforms how you relate to thought in several ways:

- Making thought is what your mind was created to do, and that is not a problem.

- Sitting with your mind as it is allows you to get familiar (and more comfortable) with having a range of thoughts without immediately reacting to them.

- You can both have thoughts and remain present in your body.

- Recognize when you have become absorbed in thought and are no longer feeling the breath in the present moment.

- Release thoughts back into the stream of consciousness gently, precisely, and without judgment.

- All thought is "just thought," separate from who you are.

Your mind, an extension of your body, will try to make sense of the world around you. When it is confused, dysregulated, or has inadequate information, your mind will do its best—sometimes that means having thoughts that are distorted or misleading. Mindfulness helps you observe yourself thinking specific thoughts and connecting the dots between what is happening in your body and your environment, what you are feeling, how you are making sense of a situation, and what action that thought leads you to take.

When you meditate, you allow your mind to be as it is. Sitting and feeling the breath while thoughts come and go, you become very familiar with your mind. The variety and intensity of thoughts can be startling. Some feel pleasant or neutral. Others are really distressing. Some come and go in a moment. Others hang around. By staying with yourself unconditionally, you come to know the very nature of your mind.

Sometimes a thought really catches your attention and carries you away. This is also not a problem. The point of meditation is not to stop thinking or to remain in perfect control of your mind; it is to let your mind be as it is while you remain present and come back whenever you get lost. To do this you must catch yourself, acknowledge the thought that took you away, and consciously let it go. This practice creates ease in detaching from thoughts.

Letting thoughts go and coming back to the feeling of breath also emphasizes how thoughts are separate from you. No matter whether they are nice, scary, silly, cruel, or any other variety, all thought is "just thought."

Mindfulness and Neuroplasticity

Mindfulness can transform thought because of neuroplasticity, which describes how the brain reorganizes synaptic connections in response to learning or experience. Scientists have discovered you can literally change your mind and learn new things at any age!

Research has shown our ways of thinking are a kind of habit. We learned to think a certain way based on influences such as genetics, temperament, what we were explicitly taught, and what we implicitly understood. It then became easier to think in this way compared with some other way.

If you grew up with only "healthy foods" allowed, you might have learned to think candy, sugar cereals, and ice cream were dangerous and off-limits. Because this was reinforced in your environment over time, it became both easier to think of these foods this way and harder to see them as just food.

It feels easier to think familiar thoughts and difficult to think new ones because the neural pathways you travel to think habitual thoughts are more accessible. When you catch yourself going down these habitual pathways, it is possible to turn away from that familiar pathway toward uncharted territory. The only difference between the old pathways and the new ones is the number of times they have been traveled. To change your mind, you must learn how to travel those new pathways as much as or more than the old ones.

Mindfulness is a form of self-directed neuroplasticity.[19] You intentionally guide your mind away from habitual neural pathways that are harmful and self-aggressive and toward pathways that are compassionate and, I would suggest, truer. You choose the types of thoughts you wish to think and guide yourself in that direction.

Because mindfulness and meditation stabilize your nervous system and help you become less reactive, you can realize what you are thinking in real time. When you recognize yourself thinking, you can notice points at which changing direction by moving away from habitual neural pathways and toward new ones aligns with Intuitive Eating. While habitual thoughts suggest there is one way to think about a situation, mindfulness and neuroplasticity show you infinite possibilities. With a compassionate and open mind, and the belief that you are the expert of yourself, you can guide your mind when you arrive at "mental forks in the road."

Shifting from Diet Mentality to Intuitive Eating

You were not born fearing food and mistrusting your body. You were not born valuing smaller bodies over larger ones. That system of thought took hold over time as it was reinforced through different channels and sources. I'm sure you have plenty of original thoughts, but dieting thoughts didn't come from you.

You might not remember this part of the process, but diet mentality took over your mind due to neuroplasticity. And neuroplasticity is your way out!

Diet mentality is not unlike a cult: imparted from the earliest age possible and meant to reach into every corner of your life. It offers specific rules and views to live by and the illusion of certainty in exchange for compliance and blind faith. The cult of dieting provides a system of thought with which to view right and wrong, safe and dangerous, good and bad.

Some parts of this are appealing. It might feel easier to be told what to eat and what not to eat. It might be a relief to know exactly how much of something is "appropriate." Such rules and regulations can feel reassuring. But there's a catch. There's no room for flexibility, and violation of protocol can send you into a tailspin. We've learned the hard way that we are not guaranteed thinness, health, or happiness even if we follow the rules perfectly. And keeping it up eventually becomes untenable.

Becoming an Intuitive Eater requires deprogramming from the cult of dieting. You must clarify differences between scientific fact, diet mentality, and your own spontaneously arising wisdom that emerges when you trust your basically good body and no longer fear food. In questioning the monolith, everything can feel like it's crashing down. This is when a framework like the ten principles of Intuitive Eating can be a lifesaver.

MINDFUL MOMENT: Trace Diet Thoughts Back to Their Origin

Where do your unique food, body, and diet thoughts originate? Did you create them? Did you choose them? Did they spontaneously arise out of nowhere? Do they determine who you are and what you do next? Might there be more to this story? Here, you will trace one of your diet thoughts back to its origin.

Get your journal. Come into your body by taking three breaths, feeling the sensation of each inhale and exhale. When you're ready, write down one of your most common diet thoughts. Then write down all the derivative thoughts related to this one. For example, if your original thought is "carbs cause weight gain," derivative thoughts might include:

- I should restrict carbs as much as I can.

- Carbs are only for cheat days.

- I should only eat carbs with one meal a day.

- I can only eat the whole-grain version of carbohydrate foods.

- Refined carbohydrates are off-limits.

- I should choose versions of typically carbohydrate-heavy food that have been modified to contain fewer carbs.

Try to recall where you were first exposed to this thought. Was it a diet commercial? A family member? Friend? How old were you at the time? Are there any reasons you may have been particularly susceptible to this thought at that time? What was the before-and-after moment this thought entered your consciousness?

Contemplate this time in your life to assess what might have helped diet mentality take root. Imagine giving the thought back to the person or thing that imparted it to you. Close your eyes or leave them gently open: envision yourself holding the thought in your hands, reinforcing it is separate from you, and hand it back to the person or thing that gave it to you.

MINDFUL MOMENT: Who Would You Be Without That Thought?

Byron Katie is known for her radical approach to helping people separate from their thoughts. "The Work" questions the validity of thoughts, examines how certain thoughts lead to problematic behaviors, and contemplates who you would be, how you would feel, and what you would do if you did not believe that thought.[20]

Open your journal to the previous exercise. Reread the diet thought you traced back to its origin. Imagine your mind without that thought. Who would you be? How might you feel? How would you behave and what choices might you make if you did not believe this thought?

Continuing with the example above, if your original thought was "carbs cause weight gain," this contemplation might go in this direction:

Carbs don't cause weight gain. They are just another macronutrient my body needs. And they are found in foods I enjoy. If I didn't believe carbs cause weight gain, I might be able to figure out what types of carbs I really like. I might focus on my eating experiences rather than depriving myself, having negative self-talk while eating carbs, or feeling guilty for eating them. I might notice when I'm becoming satisfied when eating carbs rather than overdoing it because I feel badly about myself or I'm telling myself I won't eat them again.

Return to this exercise when you have diet thoughts that trip you up to explore what it would feel like not to believe the thought.

Jackie's Story

Jackie was a new teacher. Always the "big girl" among her peers, Jackie had many narratives about her body, how others felt about it, and how her life was impacted negatively by it. One narrative was that every time something upsetting happened between Jackie and her friends, it was because of her body. We approached this story gently because of how primary it felt. We explored influences on this story, such as how the

diet culture told Jackie her life would be better when she was thinner.
We discussed how uncomfortable she was with uncertainty; "they are
rejecting me because of my body" was preferable to "I don't know why
they are rejecting me." We acknowledged that both Jackie and her
friends are messy and imperfect and responsible for their own actions.
Mindfully, Jackie poked holes in her narrative to directly experience the
painful emotions beneath it. Jackie realized that defaulting to her story
felt easier than feeling the pain of being rejected.

MINDFUL MOMENT: Choosing Your Thoughts

The Buddha said, "All that we are is the result of what we have thought." You were programmed by diet mentality. Knowing that, you can invalidate harmful narratives and replace them with anti-diet Intuitive Eating thoughts.

In this exercise, you'll identify qualities you want to nurture in your thoughts, reframe thoughts that don't possess those qualities, and practice with specific thoughts aligned with Intuitive Eating.

Grab your journal. Take a few deep embodied breaths, focusing your attention on their sensations in your body. Write down the qualities you want to nurture in your thoughts. They may align with general values for life, such as compassion, gentleness, curiosity, pleasure, and willingness to engage with uncertainty. Other qualities might include fun, connection with others, or cultivating holistic well-being.

When you notice yourself thinking specific food and body thoughts, stop and ask yourself whether they possess the qualities you want to nourish. If yes, what specific qualities are present? If no, what qualities are present? Could you offer yourself compassion and forgiveness for changing your mind? How might you reframe the thought to enhance those desired qualities? Could you acknowledge you have been influenced to think thoughts that don't represent who you are? And could you open to thoughts more genuinely aligned with who you are?

If there are specific thoughts you would like to work with—for example, "I can accept and take care of my body at this size"—this is the place for that too. Any thoughts beginning with "I wish I could think..." are worth jotting down here.

Eliana's Story

Eliana believed she had no time to care for herself. A busy pediatric physical therapist, her work both fulfilled and drained her. She often stayed up late for a little "me time" but then overslept and rushed in the mornings to get to her first appointments. When we discussed the thought that she had no time to care for herself, and considered what thought she might replace that with to align with Intuitive Eating, Eliana recognized even an hour in the morning to read and drink coffee would change the trajectory of her day. The thought aligned with that change was "I can protect some me time in the morning."

Once she shifted her thought in that direction, other pieces of the puzzle fell into place: she got to sleep earlier, which aligned with when her body told her she needed the rest, gave her the quantity and quality of sleep she needed, and helped her wake up earlier feeling on top of her day. The space she found in the morning to enjoy her coffee and read also created more room to contemplate how she wanted to eat each day. Eliana was able to balance fitting meals and snacks into her schedule and made sure they were satisfying and enjoyable.

The thoughts you think are like a marinade for your brain. Your brain takes on whatever flavor you immerse it in. Whether diet mentality or Intuitive Eating, you must make a choice; it is not an easy one but it eventually becomes clear. Once you make that decision, you can be intentional about the thoughts you think.

What Can You Celebrate?

- What did you notice about your diet-related thoughts?

- What diet thoughts can you trace back to their origin?

- What thoughts have you decided to reframe?

- What thoughts would you like to move toward?

CHAPTER 11

Cultivating Self-Compassion

When you understand your nervous system is always working to protect you—no matter how dysfunctional your thoughts or actions may seem on the surface—it becomes a little easier to have self-compassion. When this truth is contemplated regularly and mindfully, thoughts infused with self-compassion become the secret sauce of a lifelong Intuitive Eating path.

Meditation's famous association with compassion has a scientific explanation.[7] Functional MRI studies have shown changes in the brain's insula and temporal parietal junction—regions related to the perception of emotion—contribute to greater compassion. These changes, brought about by the focused attention of mindfulness, help you feel less guarded, less separate and self-oriented, and more connected to others.

In our culture, we find it easier to extend gentleness and kindness to others than to ourselves. In the Buddhist tradition, you can only offer genuine compassion to others when you feel it for yourself. One way to bridge this gap in understanding and practice is to envision yourself as an "other," just as deserving of compassion as anyone else. Take a moment to envision someone for whom you have an uncomplicated and unconditional love, such as a child or pet. Then take the feeling that arises, hold it in your heart, and envision offering it to yourself.

Dr. Kristin Neff has researched and published extensively on the topic of self-compassion. Some of her research even details the impact of a self-compassion practice on body image and eating disorder recovery.[21] Here I review the basics of self-compassion and how they apply specifically to an Intuitive Eating practice.

Self-Compassion and Intuitive Eating

Self-compassion is the practice of self-kindness over self-judgment; an understanding of common humanity rather than a sense of isolation; and a capacity for mindfulness instead of a tendency to overidentify with thought. All three of these key components apply directly to cultivating a sustainable Intuitive Eating practice.

As long as you think you are never enough, you will be willing to purchase myriad products and services. Gail Dines—feminist scholar, sociologist, and pornography researcher—famously said at the Nova Scotia Women's Summit in 2012, "If tomorrow, women in the West woke up and decided they really liked their bodies, just think how many industries would go out of business—the cosmetics industry, the clothing industry, the diet industry, the gym industry—and then think of all the allied industries supporting those industries. So when I say capitalism is dependent on women hating themselves, I'm not exaggerating." The diet culture thrives on harsh self-judgment. Dines's statement highlights the contrast between diet mentality's harshness and self-compassion's kindness.

A classic self-compassion exercise is imagining a beloved other going through a difficult time and offering them support. Then you turn the same words, tone, and intention toward yourself. Understandably, steeped in the self-aggressive and ever-judgmental culture of dieting, this may be extremely difficult and unfamiliar. Practice is key and starts with simply noticing how hard it feels to give yourself the same grace. You can even have compassion for yourself because it's so difficult to have compassion for yourself!

Recognizing how many of us are impacted by the diet culture can make it a little easier to offer ourselves that essential kindness. You have probably suffered so much of the diet culture's impact in isolation, feeling as if you were the only one struggling. But the reality is this suffering is immense and widespread. The fact that my colleagues and I do the work we do is evidence.

The things we feel most isolated about are literally the most universal: the appearance, smells, and sounds of our bodies; strong emotions such as jealousy, loneliness, or embarrassment; feelings of being different from others in distressing ways; trusting our judgment. Reminding yourself all beings suffer similarly aids in rousing compassion.

The final component of self-compassion is not overidentifying with your thoughts, not assuming your thoughts are inherently true and therefore mean something about you. Remember that analogy to describe the relationship between you and your thoughts? You are the blue sky—constant and unshakable—while thoughts are like clouds—sometimes stormy, sometimes light and fluffy, always just passing through. Applying mindfulness to your Intuitive Eating practice helps you see yourself with the same sense of constancy, without being defined by your thoughts.

Mathilde's Story

Mathilde made incredible progress with Intuitive Eating but continued to struggle with her inner critic. She was paralyzed by how she imagined others were judging her and this prevented her from doing the physical activity she craved, from dating, and from regularly stocking her home with foods. It felt as though the way Mathilde spoke to herself wouldn't budge, until we decided to work through The Mindful Self-Compassion Workbook *by Kristin Neff and Christopher Germer. Each appointment, we reviewed the work Mathilde had done, how the exercises helped her transform her inner critic into a warm, unconditional, and at times fierce advocate and friend. With continued attention and practice, Mathilde began to speak to herself in a kinder and gentler way. Mathilde continues to work on this, in subtle ways, by taking care of herself through movement, food shopping, and imagining getting out there again.*

Self-Compassion Is Not Giving Up

The most common misconception about self-compassion, particularly as it applies to working with food and your body, is that it is resigning yourself to self-indulgence. I cannot tell you how many times I have heard clients say, "If I'm compassionate toward myself, I'll never do any form of movement, I'll let myself eat whatever I want. I'll never accomplish anything." In my experience, nothing could be farther from the truth.

A confusing and sad irony is that diet culture teaches you self-aggression is "motivating," and worthiness is contingent upon compliance with food and exercise rules or with simply being in a smaller body. Self-compassion, on the other hand, is unconditional. You deserve it no matter what. Working toward accepting that reality—you are unconditionally worthy—frees you up to work with your body, mind, and heart as they continually change.

Recognizing your inherent wholeness makes the effort of Intuitive Eating worth it. Practicing that most genuine form of self-love—paying attention—helps you move away from the extremes of restriction or mindless indulgence and toward a more precise meeting of your needs.

Tamara's Story

Tamara's mom took her along to Weight Watchers meetings since she was six years old. When Tamara turned thirteen, her mom suggested she start going on her own. At sixteen, Tamara's doctor prescribed her a weight-loss drug. By eighteen, Tamara was addicted to cocaine.

Once she got sober, Tamara sought to address one of the origins of her self-destructive behavior: dieting. She entered onto an Intuitive Eating path after vowing never to diet again. One of her first steps was to regulate her eating—to have breakfast, lunch, dinner, and snacks consistently—and to begin to legalize all foods. The presence of a normal amount of food in the house was initially dysregulating for Tamara. Her strategy had been to keep as little in the house so eating required a lot of effort. Despite her commitment to Intuitive Eating and unconditionally caring for her body, Tamara was struggling. She was fearful of gaining weight. She was worried about others' judgments. And her mom was concern-trolling about Tamara's health. She felt trapped between a rock and a hard place.

We discussed the importance of being right where you are in this process, releasing attachment to thoughts, and practicing self-compassion. Tamara crafted the mantra "I know this is the right path for me and it's also really hard" to say silently or out loud to herself whenever she bumped up against the many challenges of Intuitive Eating. Continuing to offer herself kindness instead of judgment for struggling, recalling she was not alone, and working with herself honestly and without overidentifying with each fleeting thought were enough to keep Tamara going.

Practicing Self-Compassion

Intuitive Eating is innately self-compassionate. It trusts and believes in your intelligence, self-awareness, and judgment. It knows you are doing your best and that even when you do things that seem harmful or dysfunctional, you are just trying to feel safe. It understands that when you build a foundation of kindness, interconnectedness, and mindfulness you are capable of change.

A wonderfully simple way to practice self-compassion has three steps:

1. Acknowledge suffering

2. Normalize your experience

3. Offer kindness

Following these steps allows you to take the next intuitive step to address what is really going on in your body, mind, and heart.

MINDFUL MOMENT: Create Your Own Self-Compassion Statement

Grab your journal. Following the steps above, create your own self-compassion statement acknowledging whatever is causing you suffering currently, normalizing your experience in the context of the larger diet culture, and offering yourself kindness no matter what.

Here's an example of one I use from time to time:

Acknowledge suffering: "This is really hard for me. My body is hurting a lot right now. I'm still learning how to tolerate and work with chronic pain."

Normalize it: "Many people struggle with chronic pain and with tolerating discomfort. Pain does not mean I've done anything wrong. No one ever talks about this stuff. No wonder it's hard."

Offer kindness: "I am committed to keep learning to work with my life and my body as they are. I am inherently deserving of gentleness, including from myself."

Return to this mindful moment and craft a self-compassion statement to address whatever struggles you are working with as you progress on your Intuitive Eating path.

You'll need self-compassion every step of the way of your Intuitive Eating practice. From ensuring you are eating enough to ultimately healing body image, self-compassion is infused through thoughts to transform how you speak to yourself. It is what changes your internal self-talk from harsh and aggressive to kind, clear-seeing, and wise. And a self-compassion practice allows you to see yourself in all of your sweetness, vulnerability, and best intentions. It is self-compassion that reassures you: even if not everything is okay, you are okay.

What Can You Celebrate?

- In what ways has your understanding of self-compassion evolved?

- How are you beginning to work self-compassion into your self-talk?

- What did you develop as a self-compassion statement?

CHAPTER 12

Transforming Specific Diet Mentality Thoughts

Using the concepts and tools described in the last two chapters, the following list of common diet mentality thoughts are transformed to be self-compassionate and compatible with Intuitive Eating. Feel free to "use my voice" when shifting your own thoughts and know ultimately this wisdom will come directly from you.

"I can only do Intuitive Eating after I lose a little weight."

I get why this is so tempting. The diet culture has convinced you that being in a smaller body is the right thing to do on every level and worth whatever cost it exacts from your life. Yet, you know dieting doesn't work and, worse, it causes physical and mental suffering. This is such a difficult choice but please know it must be a clear choice. There is no way to have it both ways. Either choose the path of Intuitive Eating by letting your intelligent body determine what and when and how much to eat and move and by allowing your body to determine at what weight it settles. Or continue down the path of dieting (even though the diet culture will try to make it seem like it's different) with restriction, possibly bingeing, and constantly questioning yourself, because of the unlikely chance you might lose some weight.

If you choose to continue dieting, the mainstream culture will celebrate you because "at least you are making an effort to be smaller." This can feel good and supportive, but it doesn't last. If you choose Intuitive Eating, please be compassionate and gentle with yourself. Not only are you choosing to do something that is still counter to our culture, which can make it lonely, but you will also have to learn to be with yourself at whatever weight your body determines is right. If you do choose this path, know it is the last choice you ever have to make about caring for your body. More and more resources are emerging to help you stay connected to your Intuitive Eating practice and to respect and accept the body you're in. You are much more likely to enjoy your relationship with food, movement, and your life in general because how you engage with these things is based on trust, compassion, and presence.

"I can only commit to Intuitive Eating if it will help me lose weight."

When you become an Intuitive Eater, you eat primarily for physical reasons, you give yourself unconditional permission to eat, you learn to cope with strong emotions in different ways (in addition to sometimes soothing with food), and you make food choices based on what feels good in your unique and ever-changing body. Eating regularly and consistently, choosing foods that satisfy, and developing a movement practice that works for you makes you less likely to binge and so your body can work as it is meant to. All of this allows your body to settle at a weight that works for your biology. This number tends to change as you move through different ages and stages, but it is a misconception created by the diet culture that you can manipulate your weight. Weight is determined primarily by genetics and other factors out of your individual control and secondarily by the behaviors you engage in on a regular basis over time.

We don't know where your weight will settle when you become an Intuitive Eater. I know this level of uncertainty is uncomfortable. Diets are tempting because they promise you certainty that doesn't exist (but, oh, how we like to think it does!). Accepting and working with uncertainty gets a little easier when you practice meditation and mindfulness, gradually learning to tolerate more discomfort, staying present with your full experience, and taking care of yourself in real time. While you can't control your body weight, you can influence how you think about these things. Acknowledging the discomfort in not knowing, making space for the pain of living in a culture that tells you the most valuable attributes are beauty and thinness, and connecting with your tender and basically good heart and body are how you work with these realities.

"I'm not healthy at this weight."

This is such a common and strong belief. It makes sense because you get it from every angle: doctors, media, "concerned" family members. Like most things related to health, this is complex. Scientific data show us intentional efforts at weight loss are unsustainable for most, contribute to weight gain in the long run, increase disordered eating behaviors, and cause severe health problems (often misattributed to being in a larger body).

Your well-being is the most important thing. But it is not determined by weight, no matter who says it is. Trying to lose weight is not the answer. What can improve your health, however, is health-promoting behaviors: eating nutritious foods, creating a sustainable movement practice, engaging in preventive medical care, managing stress, and getting adequate quality and quantity of sleep are associated with improved laboratory measures of physical health and subjective measures of mental health.

It is scary to think your body is putting you at risk of sickness or death. At the same time, this thought is workable. When it does arise, remember you are conditioned to think it. It is not inherently true. Scientific facts and your lived experience tell you dieting does not work. Connect with the part of you that just wants to feel safe and okay. Remind that part you have all the tools necessary to enact the behaviors that improve health and that if you need additional support it exists in the form of people trained in Intuitive Eating, the *Intuitive Eating Workbook,* and online support groups.

The final thing to recall here is if you were to develop a health condition, it does not mean you did anything wrong or didn't do something you should have. The diet mentality says your health is completely within your control and anything bad that happens is your own fault. Not only is this misinformed, but it is also inhumane and misleading and causes great suffering.

"My body hurts because of my weight."

No one wants to feel pain. You are hardwired to avoid it. The truth is all bodies hurt sometimes. And pain is not doled out equitably. Some bodies feel little pain while others hurt a lot. This is a difficult truth to sit with but it can help you rouse self-compassion.

The diet culture teaches you that pain is your own fault. This is especially true if you are in a larger body. Even though different forms of pain such as back and knee pain occur at similar rates in larger bodies and smaller ones, the prevailing advice when someone in a larger body complains of pain is to lose weight.

You have options in managing your pain. Physical therapy, medication (which is not a failure), injections, strength training, cardio exercise, and meditation can all help improve your subjective experience of pain. So too does adequate quality and quantity of sleep, managing stress, treating unaddressed physical or mental health issues, and doing things that bring you joy. Pain is a mind-body experience and you are more likely to relieve it with the approaches above than by feeling badly about yourself and attempting to shrink your body.

"I don't feel like myself at this weight."

This is such a tender and vulnerable thought. It feels as if your body has betrayed you and does not represent who you are as a person. This thought comes from years and years of compounded diet mentality and weight stigma tying your worth and identity to the size and shape of your body.

The truth is *your body does not represent who you are as a person*. It could never capture the depth and expansiveness of your humanness, kindness, curiosity, suffering, and joy. What your body does do is protect you, enable you to live your life, show love, and allow you to experience the physical pleasures and pains of what it means to be human.

Think of your whole self—body, mind, heart, and soul. What are the various pieces of the puzzle: your relationships, passions, profession, worldview? Where does your body fit in? What proportion of your life is occupied by your body and does that represent your values? Can you zoom out and appreciate how the diet culture teaches you to fixate on a relatively small piece of your whole self with extreme criticism and negativity? Can you imagine a mind-set in which your body assumes its rightful place as part of your life and experience, as something that sometimes feels pain or causes suffering but also brings great joy and engagement with your life?

"I don't feel hungry until I'm starving."

Before you are in the habit of noticing, interpreting, and responding to subtle sensations of hunger it's common not to recognize it until it's extreme. Whether due to a history of ignoring or mistrusting hunger signals, eating sporadically, habitually restricting, and/or bingeing, you may find it difficult to recognize hunger before it becomes urgent and primal.

How to work with this thought:

- Review the various signs of hunger and assess which ones seem to arise in your body.

- Use a temporary structured approach to eating at regular intervals and welcome hunger signals.

- Assess whether anything might be interfering with sensing hunger, such as medications, poor sleep, stress, or untreated physical or mental illness.

You may also have an entrenched belief you only "deserve" to eat once you are extremely hungry. By giving yourself permission to eat when gently hungry and observing what kind of eating experience you have when you do so, you provide the evidence needed to practice this more frequently.

"I know when I'm comfortably full, but I can't stop eating until I'm in pain."

As you learned in the chapter on fullness, this part of your Intuitive Eating path should be approached with gentleness and discernment. Because most of your dieting life was focused on stopping eating as early as possible, it will take time to feel stopping when comfortably full is self-care.

Recognizing when you are full is good news! That means you have honed interoception to sense and interpret sensations of comfortable fullness. Even though it is clear when you are comfortably full physically, you may not have reached the point of emotional satisfaction that feels like "enough."

It sounds like there is something missing for you when you get to this point. Do you suspect you won't have access to the food again? Are you still working on unconditional permission to eat? Are you permitting yourself to eat the foods you find most satisfying? Are there other unmet needs in your life that you haven't figured out yet?

Whatever the reason, it is okay! Be right where you are and know you will get there with time. Continue to notice when you reach comfortable fullness and ask yourself what is going on in those moments—physically, mentally, and emotionally. Eventually you will reach a point when you feel both full and satisfied and when choosing to stop eating feels as accessible as choosing to continue.

"Stopping when I'm full feels like restriction."

After a long history of restriction, this makes sense. Your body and mind still fear deprivation. You feel an urgent need to eat as much as you can, even if that means a less pleasurable eating experience when your body is full and you keep eating. Continue eating regularly and satisfyingly, finding a balance of protein, carbohydrate, and fat. Continue reinforcing your unconditional permission to eat, prioritizing your personal satisfaction. Continue tending to your emotional needs for pleasure, rest, connection, fun, and intimacy so it is clear when you need food to soothe and when you need something else. You will get there eventually.

Coming to the end of a pleasurable experience is often sad or disappointing. Eating is pleasurable, so reaching the end of a meal doesn't feel as good as the beginning. What if you were to acknowledge when you are full, assess your residual drive to eat, and consider whether you feel ready to sit with the sadness and/or disappointment of stopping? Your mindfulness practice supports you in tolerating such moderate discomfort. You might not look forward to the end of meals, but you might start to feel less distressed about them.

"I eat whenever I get the urge (even if I'm not hungry) because saying no feels like restriction."

Similar to difficulty stopping when comfortably full, it is common to always eat when you get the urge, when food is offered to you, or when the opportunity suddenly arises. When you were dieting, the answer was always "no." Even if you ate in those circumstances, you were probably thinking, "I shouldn't be eating this," which is just like saying no except with a side order of guilt.

As long as you continue to eat regularly and avoid the danger zone of hunger, and as long as you eat the foods you want and reinforce unconditional permission to eat, you will eventually reach a point where saying "no" feels less threatening.

This requires your attention, patience, and compassion. Saying "yes" when your body doesn't need food is not different from saying "no" when it does. Neither meets your body's true needs. There is nothing wrong with choosing to eat when you are not hungry (though it *is* wrong to not eat when you are hungry). A peaceful relationship with food includes being able to say "no" in an uncomplicated way when your internal wisdom tells you food is not what's needed.

"But sugar/carbs/processed foods *are* bad for me."

The current manifestation of the diet culture, which purports to be rooted in health promotion, is so confusing on this issue. It tells you there are certain foods you shouldn't eat, not because they'll make you fat (but they do suggest this is also true), but because they can make you sick. Sugar, carbohydrates, and processed and packaged foods are the present-day public enemies like fat, saturated fat, and cholesterol were in the 1990s. Like all things, there is a lot more to this story than it seems.

Your body adapts to whatever you throw at it. If you consume too much of most vitamins and minerals, for example, it excretes what it doesn't need. If you don't consume enough, it will use what it does have more efficiently. The body's detoxification system—liver, kidneys, skin, and lungs—work to keep you healthy and free from dangerous levels of certain chemicals (remember, everything is chemicals, even us!). Even if your diet contains processed and packaged foods, added sugars, and carbohydrate-containing foods, it will not threaten your health.

What *can* threaten your health is the level of stress when you think that food is dangerous and you have to be hypervigilant to protect yourself. Eating while stressed contributes to poor health, robs you of joy, causes self-doubt, and might paradoxically lead you to eat more of these "fearsome" foods than you would if they were just part of a varied diet.

"But eating salt, sugar, and fat overrides my ability to sense fullness and satisfaction."

Do food companies conduct research to determine the exact amount of salt, sugar, and fat is the most palatable? Yes. Was there a semi-famous scientist who claimed that because of this, most people are not capable of mindful eating? Yes, but much of his data were fabricated and he has been defrocked in the nutrition science community. Does your "mindful eating equipment" still work in the face of extremely palatable foods? Also yes.

A varied diet—which is the diet 100 percent of my clients develop by staying on the path of Intuitive Eating—can and should contain foods so delicious they make your head spin a little. The point of not getting too hungry and routinely eating the foods you want is you hone detection of sensory-specific satiety, that point at which food starts to taste a little less spectacular. This happens even for the tastiest foods. Bring your full attention to these eating experiences and acknowledge when you get lost in thoughts that you shouldn't be eating them or that they alter your ability to eat mindfully. Keep coming back to that sensory experience and notice what your body communicates.

"I'm addicted to sugar/carbs."

Oooof, shoddy science has been hard at work jamming this idea down our throats. I'm sure you've seen the functional MRIs of "a brain on sugar" alongside "a brain on heroin" or other addictive substance. Because sugar lights up the pleasure centers in the brain, we are meant to believe it is no different from heroin. Really? But these studies leave out important information.

Lots of things light up the pleasure centers in the brain—a hug from someone you love, watching cat videos, or catching a beautiful sunrise. And, yes, food lights up the brain; because it is considered pleasurable, we are motivated to eat, which means we get to survive. The brain's preferred source of fuel is glucose or sugar. If your body does not get it, compensatory mechanisms built into your biology increase your desire and seeking behavior for it.

Those studies (which are mostly done in rat models) do not control for the effects of restriction. If you don't give sugar to a study subject—rat or human—and then give them unlimited access, they very well might overdo it. But if given consistent access to these foods, there is no rebound bingeing. You have probably experienced this for yourself. If you believe sugar is addictive and tried to restrict it, you may have reached a point where you couldn't resist anymore and binged on sugar. This would have confirmed you were indeed addicted, which strengthened your resolve to restrict, and on and on.

"I'm craving salad/greens/fruit...does that mean I'm moving back toward dieting?"

This is such a common concern, but I'll tell you why it's usually good news: when you give yourself unconditional permission to eat and listen to your body, heart, and mind, all foods find their place on the same moral plane. No foods are good or bad, condoned or off-limits. Every client I have worked with through early challenges of Intuitive Eating has eventually craved a varied diet. That means in addition to the once-charged foods you normalize, you are drawn to foods you previously ate out of a sense of obligation to your diet.

Maybe you had to take a break from these foods to gain perspective. That is a great way to respect where you are in the process and trust that your wisdom will ultimately guide you toward what you need. The fact that you're craving what you once thought of as "healthy" foods tells me you have moved through a phase of Intuitive Eating in which you feel pressured to eat a certain way and your intuition for what will taste good and feel good in your body is emerging.

"I can't separate movement from dieting/weight loss."

Please be patient with this part of the process. You may never have had the experience of moving your body just because it feels good. The conditioning around exercise as a means of earning your calories or managing your weight is so deeply ingrained and it will take patience, time, and experimentation to reframe.

Thinking you cannot separate movement from dieting may indicate you are not quite ready to create a movement practice. You are still healing from the damage done by the diet culture where exercise was a punishing obligation. This might be time to explore your past with movement, not just as a dieter but before then.

If you can recall when movement was enjoyable, what was that like? How did it feel? What part of it would you like to feel again? If you cannot recall such a time, imagine how you would like to feel about a movement practice. Try to let go of the expectation to "jump on the movement wagon" and consider this a time of contemplation and spaciousness. You will get there.

"I don't know how to feed myself."

Whenever I hear this, I think it is a form of amnesia caused by fear. You might be afraid Intuitive Eating is too much for you or there's something different about your body that makes it impossible. This is simply not true. You can do this and this thought is providing an opportunity to engage with yourself compassionately, with an open and flexible mind.

When this thought arises, connect with a framework, something that feels supportive and reliable to you. This may be a structured approach to eating regular meals each day (see chapter 3 for details). This may be the three-step approach to rousing self-compassion: acknowledging suffering, normalizing your suffering, offering yourself kindness (see chapter 11 for more on this).

This is also an opportunity to return to your journal and review your "noticings," celebrations, and accomplishments. This is exactly why you record them, so they are there when you need them. If you do this, commemorate this moment too: record how you were questioning whether you know how to feed yourself, and then you remembered there was a repository of examples of how you do exactly that.

"I can't sustain this."

This sounds like you're doing something that feels too hard to keep up long term. I wonder whether the fear of not sustaining an Intuitive Eating practice comes from the belief that it must be perfect and look the same each day. You may be looking at Intuitive Eating through the lens of diet mentality in which there are finite and specific goals and rules you must comply with day in and day out. That is not the case with Intuitive Eating. The uncertainty inherent in Intuitive Eating is what makes it so liberating, but it can also feel more difficult at first.

How would it feel to take a one-day-at-a-time approach? You don't need to have everything figured out. Take care of your human body and tender heart. Come back to the basics of prioritizing sleep, not going longer than four hours without eating, eating a balance of protein and carbohydrate and fat, drinking enough water, and managing stress. Determine whether there is fun, rest, pleasure, and connection in your life. When the thought that you cannot sustain an Intuitive Eating practice arises, acknowledge this as suffering, normalize that it takes time to adjust to a completely new way of being in the world, and offer yourself the kindness of asking, "What am I feeling right now and what do I truly need to feel okay?"

"I think about food too much."

When people start Intuitive Eating after years of dieting, restriction, and confusion, they might think the goal is to stop thinking about food. This is not realistic because we all need to think about food sometimes: shopping for it, preparing it, what restaurant to go to, checking in with how food is tasting, and so on. What seems to make a difference is *how* you are thinking about food.

At the beginning, it is not uncommon to think about food a lot and in an obsessive way. You may fixate on all the ways you want to change your relationship with food and believe the more you focus on them, the quicker they will change. Unfortunately, this doesn't seem to be true. My guidance on working with food thoughts is to understand the typical progression and then see where you are.

A typical progression is to begin with obsessive thought and then gradually move toward what I call "hyperawareness." Different from obsession, hyperawareness may feel like a similar amount of thoughts, but the quality of those thoughts is more concerned with noticing and making connections. As you continue to be hyperaware and you understand connections between beliefs, thoughts, feelings, and behaviors around food, your thinking will gradually shift toward "mindfulness." Mindfulness gives you real-time awareness so that, even if something doesn't feel good, it doesn't feel as distressing as when you were obsessive.

The bottom line is to trust yourself and the process, have patience, and continue to speak to yourself with compassion.

"I can't change at this point in my life."

This is such a natural fear. How many times have you heard the expression "You can't teach an old dog new tricks"? Yet neuroplasticity tells us you can indeed teach an old dog new tricks. It is a gradual and cumulative process of noticing habitual thoughts, catching yourself at some point and choosing to proceed in a different (even if only slightly different) direction, and then assessing whether that course correction felt better for you.

Mindfulness and meditation stabilize body and mind so you can observe yourself in real time rather than realizing what happened in retrospect. Self-compassion helps you speak to yourself gently, normalize your suffering, and feel less isolated. This is how change happens. At any stage of life.

"I used to feel a connection with Intuitive Eating, but I've lost it and I can't get it back."

This path is not a straight line. Even in the best of circumstances, ups and downs are normal with Intuitive Eating. Real life feels no obligation to remain in the best of circumstances, especially during a global pandemic that stretches on for years. Could you give yourself permission to have an Intuitive Eating practice that is messy and imperfect but also flexible and attuned? Could you give yourself permission not to be perfectly consistent all the time, to need breaks, to come back after a little while?

That you have decided to stop dieting and learn how to have a peaceful, satisfying, and joyful relationship with food and your body suggests you are already an Intuitive Eater. An Intuitive Eater who continues to learn how to be with themself through life's twists and turns. You may be in a period of your life when things feel less clear. Can you use this time to come back to the basics, meeting your most foundational physical and emotional needs and assessing whether there are any gaps? Can you double down on your self-compassion practice and reassure yourself you are unconditionally deserving of grace, forgiveness, and gentleness? This is how you move through life as an Intuitive Eater.

With mindfulness and compassion, all thought becomes workable. Change is possible when you see where you are and stay with your experience. Your meditation practice helps you do just that with openness, tenderness, and maybe even a sense of humor.

What Can You Celebrate?

- What diet mentality thoughts are you currently working with?

- What diet mentality thoughts have you already worked through?

- What did you learn about responding to harmful thoughts with compassion and curiosity?

- What are you excited to try?

PART IV

Mindfulness of Phenomena

With mindfulness of phenomena, your relationship with food and your body speaks to your relationship with life on a larger scale. The microscopic ways you relate to food and your body speak volumes about how you *are* in your life. Once you see this, you can work with it.

With constancy of attention—to the physical body, emotions, and thoughts—you maintain an expansive and panoramic view of your life. Suffering, impermanence, and egolessness are enduring truths; accepting them gives you access to delight, joy, and an embodied life.

Through constant change, with all manner of discomfort, and by acknowledging your interconnectedness with others, you are capable of so much more than pathologizing who and how you are. This leads to powerful change in the world.

CHAPTER 13

How You Do Anything Is How You Do Everything

There is a saying: "How you do anything is how you do everything." I'm not sure who said it first, but it feels very true. My work with clients and my own personal experiences have shown me that how you engage with the different aspects of your life demonstrates your basic view about the way things are. Whether or not you are conscious of this specific view, it finds its way into every part of your life.

When my view was governed by grasping onto pleasure and avoiding pain—not making any mistakes—that is what showed up in my relationships, my profession, and my thinking about the future. I was anxious, self-doubting, rarely content, and often felt I was missing something everyone else had figured out. When mindfulness and meditation taught me about the inevitability of suffering and the preciousness of the present moment, that view shaped my relationship with food and my body, my love life, motherhood, work, and friendships. Everything started to feel workable, tender, and poignant. "Getting it right" became a useless concept distracting me from what mattered.

The underlying view of both mindfulness and Intuitive Eating includes:

- Working with things as they are

- Remaining present, flexible, and gentle

- Respecting your innate intelligence and goodness

Relating to food and your body through Intuitive Eating and mindfulness becomes the practice ground for these foundational views. Eating and relating to your body with this view helps you open to uncertainty, discomfort, pleasure, and delight. Ultimately this becomes how you live your life.

Many of my clients have discovered how their relationship with food revealed important insights about how they relate to life in general: relationships, work, pleasure and fun, sensuality and sex, conflict, discomfort, uncertainty, and change. Look to your relationship with food for insights on how you relate to your body, to other flawed humans, to your environment, and to the larger world of phenomena. Intuitive Eating and mindfulness guide you—through your work on food and body—to bring the elements of presence, flexibility, and gentleness to the rest of your life.

This chapter shares some insights into bringing the underlying view of Intuitive Eating and mindfulness into your life, specifically in the areas of:

- Pleasure

- Well-being

- Social justice

- Acceptance

- Everyday magic

Notice if you see yourself here.

Pleasure

Pleasure can be complicated. You might have fears, judgments, negative connotations, or a general mistrust of pleasure. Considering the influence of both the diet culture and prevailing Judeo-Christian beliefs in the West, that is not surprising. Their consensus is pleasure can be dangerous or shameful. And this might have led you to deprioritize pleasure, to deny your desires, or to engage in pleasurable activities only secretly, sheepishly, and with a sense of guilt.

And yet pleasure is so deeply human. Taste, smell, touch, hearing, and sight—how could pleasuring these senses be wrong? Your senses enable you to connect with your own body, with other bodies, and with your environment in ways that bring richness, depth, and sensuality. In a word: life.

The senses exist only in the present moment; that makes connecting with them the most mindful—and human—activity you can engage in. Prioritizing pleasure, focusing on what brings your senses the most appealing, joyful, or even blissful experience, can become a regular practice of anchoring into the present moment. Focusing on pleasure sharpens mindfulness; feeling pleasure helps you stay in the present moment and recognize when you've gotten lost so you can come back. Some added motivation to prioritize pleasure: it feels really good!

In her book *Pleasure Activism: The Politics of Feeling Good,* adrienne maree brown positions pleasure as a radical daily practice. She even suggests having an orgasm before diving into each new section of her book as a means of connecting with your body and the practice of pleasure. Challenging its traditional position as an afterthought—especially for women and marginalized communities who experience disproportionately high stress and trauma—pleasure must be pursued intentionally, directly, and possibly to the detriment of others' needs, at least initially. This is about putting yourself first.

Not surprisingly, brown was deeply influenced by the work of Audre Lorde, whose famous essay "The Uses of the Erotic: The Erotic as Power" first suggested the potency and power of self-love for women. Lorde writes, "The erotic is a measure between the beginnings of our sense of self and the chaos of our strongest feelings. It is an internal sense of satisfaction to which, once we have experienced it, we know we can aspire." Lorde positions pleasure not as something solely self-indulgent but a spiritual practice so self-reverent it benefits the individual and everyone around her.

Self-compassion researcher Kristin Neff also emphasizes the power of pleasure in her supportive touch meditation. In this practice, you simply place your hand on your own heart, stroke your arm, or cradle your face in your hands to soothe your vulnerable self through physical touch. Pleasure here is the conduit for self-compassion.

Supportive touch was a particularly important meditation for many of my clients who struggled with the loss of intimacy and physical touch during the pandemic. Many questioned the idea of offering themselves supportive touch at first. Yet their ability to physically soothe their bodies with pleasurable touch was so basic, pure, and readily available. Those who practiced it have another coping skill in their toolbox.

Another oft-underused form of pleasure is rest. Rest is not just getting your eight hours of sleep a night. It is napping and/or restoring somehow with your eyes open throughout the day. Feeling you need to earn rest is no less toxic than feeling you need to earn your calories. The Nap Ministry was founded by Tricia Hersey as an organization that examines the liberating power of naps. Their "rest is resistance" framework—created specifically for women of color—explores the restorative practice of napping by contrast with the grind culture.

Intuitive Eating coupled with mindfulness can be an entry point into a pleasure practice. You have already learned centering pleasure and satisfaction fuels your body's inborn self-regulation. Not only does emphasizing preferred tastes, temperatures, and textures please your senses, but it also enables you to recognize sensations of the rise and dissolution of pleasure within an eating experience. Pleasure helps you feed yourself with a new degree of precision.

Pleasure is also emphasized in a sustainable movement practice. Focusing attention on the somatic experience and the joy inherent in moving, you reorient your relationship with movement toward enjoyment. You can finally ask, *How would I like to move my body? What feels good to me? What do I like to do?* Elevating pleasure draws you into movement not as an obligation but as an expression of self-love.

Building on the foundation introduced by Intuitive Eating and mindfulness, and to make pleasure an intentional practice, consider the following questions:

- How do I spend my time? How much of this is motivated by pleasure?

- What do I look at? What books, films, TV shows, artworks, and natural landscapes light up my brain's pleasure centers?

- What do I listen to? What music, podcasts, broadcasts, spoken word, audiobooks, and nature sounds draw me in and fill me up?

- How do I dress myself? Does this give me joy and comfort? Is it fun? How could it become more fun?

- How do I care for my body, and which aspects are particularly pleasurable?

- Who do I spend time with? With whom do I laugh? Connect? Dream?

- How do I feel in my relationships? What brings me pleasure in connecting with others?

- How am I giving and/or receiving sensual pleasure?

- What is my relationship with my sexuality? How do I connect with my sexual self?

- How do I recharge? Do I prefer restful or invigorating activities?

- What do I do for fun? How do I engage with creativity, music, art, fashion, film, nature, games, sports, play, or anything else that brings me joy?

- What makes me laugh, and how often do I access those things? How could I laugh more?

- How am I actively addressing the barriers to prioritizing and practicing pleasure in my life?

MINDFUL MOMENT: Then and Now: What Was/Is Your Relationship with Pleasure?

In this exercise, you will be contemplating your relationship with pleasure when you were dieting and since beginning your Intuitive Eating and mindfulness practices.

Grab your journal. Try to recall what connotations you had about pleasure when you were dieting. How did that affect your thoughts about pleasure? How did that affect how you pursued pleasure? How often did you ask yourself the following questions:

- What tastes would give me pleasure?

- What sounds give me goosebumps?

- What kinds of touch or texture make my eyes roll back in my head?

- What smells and aromas give me joy?

- What can I look at that would fill me with delight?

- What would feel good to me right now?

- What could I do for fun today?

- How can I bring more pleasure into my life?

If you did ask any of these questions, did you pursue that pleasure?

Now review the questions from where you feel you are now. As an Intuitive Eater and mindfulness and meditation practitioner, what is your current relationship with pleasure? What are the sources of pleasure in your life and how do you relate to them? How do you answer the questions above?

Well-Being

Well-being is another area of life reflected in your relationship with food and your body. When you were dieting, I imagine there was a straight line between thinness and wellness, and by extension another straight line between ill health and allowing your body to be as it is. Your definition of well-being, therefore, may have been an oversimplified iteration of "lose weight to be well."

The size of your body does not determine your well-being. Not even a little. That misinformation is part and parcel of the diet culture sham placing the full responsibility of well-being on you. The myth is you control your own health destiny and therefore your well-being is under your control. This is how the medical institution and diet culture–adjacent industries justify subpar care and services for people in larger bodies.

The truth is the predominant causes of health outcomes are out of our control: genetics and social determinants of health such as education, economic stability, safety of your environment, social infrastructure, and access to nutritious food and quality health care. Your health is not your fault. If you develop type 2 diabetes, for example, it is not because of something you did or didn't do. There were likely several confluent factors, many completely out of your control, culminating in insulin resistance and irregular glucose control.

In joining the Intuitive Eating movement, particularly when you do so with the attunement of a mindfulness practice, you see the holes in the weight-equals-health myth. You see yourself as the only true expert of yourself. And you recognize well-being is subjective: you get to define it. Is well-being a priority? What does well-being look like for you? (Some people have been so harmed by the health care system that they need to deprioritize "health" to heal that trauma.)

Once you consult your values and wisdom to define well-being, you can turn toward the behaviors you do have control over: movement, eating the nutritious foods you do have access to, engaging in preventive health care, getting adequate quantity and quality of sleep, reducing stress, taking your medications as prescribed, and tending to your mental health. When you engage with health-promoting behaviors from a place of agency—with power and resources to support you—rather than learned helplessness, guilt, and shame, you are more likely to sustain them and feel good about your self-care.

True well-being is holistic: an intersection of physical, mental, social, environmental, and spiritual factors. Some aspects are grand and sweeping, others are microscopic and boring. Setting boundaries and defending them—an often-invisible part of self-care—is just as important as advocating for yourself in the health care system and seeking out providers who are compatible with Intuitive Eating. Declining to be weighed unless it is medically necessary is as important as emphasizing the real parameters of physical well-being, such as blood glucose levels, blood pressure, cholesterol and triglycerides, liver function tests, and thyroid hormones.

Choosing the foods that make your body feel good becomes just as important as choosing foods that please your taste buds. Both become intentional expressions of self-care and self-love. So too does putting yourself first, even if that is an inconvenient change for some of the people in your life. It's one thing for your loved ones to want you to care for yourself, and another for them to be willing to be inconvenienced when you do so. Let others take the hit once in a while!

Some individuals who have reframed wellness through their writing, business offerings, and health-related practices include:

- Jessamyn Stanley, yoga teacher and author of *Every Body Yoga* and *Yoke: My Yoga of Self-Acceptance*

- Roz "the Diva" Mays, personal trainer, pole diva, and star of the documentary *Dangerous Curves*

- Bethany Meyers, fitness entrepreneur and CEO of the be.come project

- Gloria Lucas, founder and CEO of Nalgona Positivity Pride

MINDFUL MOMENT: What Is Your Emerging Definition of Well-Being?

In your journal, explore your emerging definition of well-being as the result of your Intuitive Eating and mindfulness practices. What does well-being mean to you today? What does it encompass? What does it intentionally leave out? Where does it diverge from the mainstream culture's definition of well-being? Return to this mindful moment whenever you realize another layer of your own definition of well-being—and know it will always be emerging.

Social Justice

When you make pleasure a practice, when you create your own vision of well-being, you realize everyone deserves the same. When you accept and work with your body as it is, you relate to others as whole and deserving of love, compassion, kindness, support, inclusion, access, visibility, and dignity. There is an inherent connection between Intuitive Eating, mindfulness, and respect for all bodies, and between respect for all bodies and social justice efforts to make whole-person well-being equitably available to all.

Staggering disparities prevent everyone from living peaceably, safely, and well. By rejecting the diet culture, you see how the world has justified neglecting bodies that don't fit the preferred profile: fat bodies, normal bodies, most bodies. We discover the diet culture is not an innocuous social construct fueled by health or vanity. It is deeply flawed, biased, and dangerous. In her book *Fearing the Black Body: The Racial Origins of Fat Phobia*, Sabrina Strings highlights connections between the idealization of thinness and the idealization of whiteness. Participating in and benefiting from the diet culture upholds this inhumane dynamic. Dismantling it is the only option.

This is where Intuitive Eating and mindfulness as "self-help techniques" become activism. The underlying view of meditation was never about self-improvement, but about being of benefit to others. By confirming your own basic goodness and intelligence, by creating a practice of presence and compassion, you ultimately bring more compassion and sanity into the world. The individual work you do with Intuitive Eating already contributes to a more just world. Often, though, Intuitive Eaters discover the motivation to bring this sanity beyond the boundaries of their own bodies.

This initially shows up in small ways. To feed yourself according to your wisdom and needs, you must quiet the voices that interfere. Those voices don't just exist in your own head. Messages from the people in your home and workplace may elicit self-doubt, shame, and confusion around food and body. Comments are made thoughtlessly around the dinner table. Changes in your body are noticed out loud. Family members or coworkers you once enlisted as the diet police might need to be told their services are no longer needed. Perhaps instead you wish to redirect them to support your new self-compassionate approach to eating. In each of these scenarios, you might need to assert your needs unapologetically and have some difficult conversations. Doing this plants seeds of awareness, openness, and curiosity instead of allowing ignorance to flourish. And you are taking skillful action.

Establishing and defending boundaries, teaching family, friends, and health care providers how you expect to be treated and spoken to, placing your own mental and physical well-being above that of others—this is how you step into the role of activist with Intuitive Eating. These actions might also give rise to larger examples: voting with your wallet to support fashion brands catering to real bodies, voting with your actual vote to make health care more accessible across social demographics, doing research to understand your own role in upholding unjust systems, and actively engaging as a changemaker.

This capacity for change comes from your ability to stay with discomfort. Mindfulness has supported you to understand your difficult emotions, responses to uncertainty, and resistance to change. It also ultimately supports you to take this fierce compassion further. In his book *My Grandmother's Hands: Racialized Trauma and the Pathway to Mending Our Hearts and Bodies*, Resmaa Menakem highlights how the ability to mindfully stay with our discomfort helps us heal. He writes,

> *Healing trauma involves recognizing, accepting, and moving through pain—clean pain. It often means facing what you don't want to face—what you have been reflexively avoiding or fleeing. By walking into that pain, experiencing it fully, and moving through it, you*

metabolize it and put an end to it. In the process, you also grow, create more room in your nervous system for flow and coherence, and build your capacity for further growth.

Clean pain is about choosing integrity over fear. It is about letting go of what is familiar but harmful, finding the best parts of yourself, and making a leap—with no guarantee of safety or praise. This healing does not happen in your head. It happens in your body. And it is more likely to happen in a body that can stay settled in the midst of conflict and uncertainty.

What begins as a desire to better understand your emotional relationship with food can blossom into something we all benefit from. Your willingness and ever-expanding capacity to sit with your own discomfort ultimately makes you a powerful ally to those fighting for a more just world. In addition to Resmaa Menakem, other thought leaders exploring the connections between mindfulness and embodied social justice include:

- Michael Yellow Bird, dean and professor, faculty of social work, University of Manitoba, enrolled member of MHA (Mandan, Hidatsa, and Arikara) Nation in South Dakota, and teacher of neurodecolonization and mindfulness

- Rhonda V. Magee, mindfulness teacher and author of *The Inner Work of Racial Justice: Healing Ourselves and Transforming Our Communities Through Mindfulness*

- Lama Rod Owens, Buddhist minister, activist, yoga instructor, and author of *Radical Dharma: Talking Race, Love, and Liberation* and *Love and Rage: The Path of Liberation Through Anger*

- Gail Parker, psychologist, yoga therapy educator, and author of *Restorative Yoga for Ethnic and Race-Based Stress and Trauma* and *Transforming Ethnic and Race-Based Traumatic Stress with Yoga*

- Michelle Cassandra Johnson, race equity and anti-racism trainer, social justice warrior, yoga teacher, and author of *Skill in Action:*

Radicalizing Your Yoga Practice to Create a Just World and *Finding Refuge: Heart Work for Healing Collective Grief*

- Reverend angel Kyodo williams, Zen priest and author of *Radical Dharma: Talking Race, Love, and Liberation* and *Being Black: Zen and the Art of Living with Fearlessness and Grace*

- Ruth King, founder of the Mindful of Race Institute and author of *Mindful of Race: Transforming Racism from the Inside Out*

MINDFUL MOMENT: What Is Your Relationship with Social Justice?

Journal time. Please engage in this exercise with nonjudgmental curiosity as you reflect on the following questions. What has been your relationship with activism and social justice? In what ways have Intuitive Eating and mindfulness influenced your view of changing unjust systems? How do you see yourself enacting social justice efforts to allow yourself to live authentically, healthfully, joyously? How do you see yourself enacting behaviors that could impact others?

Acceptance

"Grant me the serenity to accept the things I cannot change, the courage to change the things I can, and the wisdom to know the difference." These words close thousands of 12-step meetings every day as people battle their demons, and the other demons they used to hush the original ones. Accepting the things we cannot change is complicated.

If I had to choose the simplest definition of mindfulness, it would be accepting reality: the way things are. Not how we wish they were, not how we believe they should be. Just as they are. We can have feelings about reality—really strong feelings of love and hatred, preference and aversion. We are not always going to like reality. That is fine. But life feels no obligation to constantly please us. So part of working with reality and ultimately accepting it is accepting our feelings about it.

When you begin an Intuitive Eating practice, you are training in acceptance. You accept your human body has needs that must be met, and fighting with those needs has many negative consequences. You accept you are inherently an emotional being deserving of compassion and you are always evolving and changing in important ways because everything is always evolving and changing. Gradually you learn to accept the reality of discomfort and tend to your deepest emotional needs in ways that don't always involve food. This is where acceptance takes root.

One of the most challenging parts of an Intuitive Eating practice is accepting the reality of the body that is adequately fed and cared for. It likely won't comply with what you have been encouraged to strive for. So where does that leave you? How do you extend your practice of acceptance to the body you live in?

The short answer is with time and patience. The longer one has many facets.

Because you were fed a steady diet of images of unattainable bodies, you must consciously and intentionally consume images that expand this perspective. Look around you, not at the bodies provoking negative comparisons, but at the real bodies that were always there. You can do a form of body exposure therapy by seeking out images of bodies that are both different from yours and similar to yours; noticing what thoughts, feelings, and sensations arise; and noticing how these change over time.

Another way to accept a broader range of bodies, including yours, is to view the work of artists who have a deep love for and curiosity about bodies. Their creative works explore the body's functionality, its humanness, its fleshy dimpled reality. Some of my favorite body-oriented artists include:

- Joan Semmel, painter

- Senga Nengudi, sculptor and visual artist

- Shoog McDaniel, photographer

- John Coplans, photographer

- Diane Arbus, photographer

- Sally Hewett, stitch and embroidery artist

- Jenny Saville, painter

- Bill T. Jones, choreographer

- Rebecca Belmore, sculpture, installation, and performance artist

- Symone, drag queen and winner of *RuPaul's Drag Race* season 13

When you observe bodies in this way, try not to focus on snap judgments of like, dislike, don't care. Instead, notice shape, line, color, texture, movement. Your raw perception, free of automatic judgment, will help you truly see what is there. Like staring into one of those Magic Eye paintings, could you see what is hidden beyond your initial impression?

Could you open to difference and become curious about it? Could you inquire deeper than appearance and consider how others' lives are affected by our collective intolerance to difference? What if we experienced life as richer and deeper by expanding to accommodate difference? What if we didn't just tolerate but sought out and celebrated difference?

As you continue on your Intuitive Eating and mindfulness path, notice when you are able to accept reality and when you are resistant to it. Use your journal to note your observations, trends, and changes over time.

MINDFUL MOMENT: Softening Resistance into Acceptance

This is a practice to do when you notice yourself struggling to accept some aspect of your life, whether your present-moment body, hurt feelings, or garden-variety anxiety or restlessness.

When you feel yourself resisting something, get your journal and lie down. Make sure you are physically comfortable, adequately fed, and well rested— basically, ensure your nervous system feels safe enough to feel some discomfort.

Close your eyes lightly or leave them gently open. Take three deep and embodied breaths, feeling the air coming in through the nose and going out through the nose. Feel where your body connects with the ground and drop in. Bring to mind the subject provoking resistance. What sensations are present in your body? Is there tension, tightness, hot or cold, pain? Let your attention rest on each area of activation or deactivation for a few moments, staying with the sensation, gently but precisely letting go of the story attached.

After spending a few moments with these sensations, choose one and see whether you might soften that area of your body. If, for example, you are experiencing pain, can you release any bracing against it? What is it like to experience just the raw sensation without adding anything to it? Spend time with the sensations once you have softened into them. Record any "noticings" in your journal.

You may or may not notice immediate changes in your cognitive resistance to what is troubling you. Continue to play with this practice in the body, and observe over time what happens.

Everyday Magic

So much of diet culture is fixated on a fantasy about how life should be, could be, if only… Intuitive Eating and mindfulness, on the contrary, focus on the immediacy of your experience: right here and now. You are alive. What are you going to do about it?

Anchored in the present moment, you might notice things you didn't before: colors, sounds, textures, tastes, subtle dynamics, sensations, fleeting thoughts. Some of these might be pleasant, others unpleasant, a lot of them neutral. It is the noticing itself that is important.

When you notice the little things, fixating less on how life should be different, there can be appreciation and gratitude. Meditation brought me a sense of reverence for my ordinary everyday life. For the tiny interactions between myself and my partner or my son (like when he called the shower pouf a "soap multiplier"…genius!), the gooey tang of my favorite cheese on the crispest crackers, the sun shining through golden leaves as I head down the driveway to school pickup. Suddenly I was surrounded by sacredness I had never noticed before.

Not that everything is great. But recognizing this everyday magic has helped me create positivity bias in my life. You might have heard of negativity bias, fixating on the problems or dangers we face as an evolutionary benefit that kept us safe. In the absence of predators, our negativity bias sometimes leads us to ignore what is good and right. Meditation increased my bias toward noticing the positive, not to the exclusion of the negative, but in a more balanced way.

Through your Intuitive Eating and mindfulness practice, what could you start to notice that you didn't before? Is it the comfort of sitting in your favorite chair at the end of the day? The texture of the fur behind your cat's ears (how can it be so soft?)? The perfect bite of peanut butter and jelly? This is the everyday magic that adds richness, wonder, and delight to your life. You don't have to wait for it. It's all around you.

The beauty of everyday magic is that it's not out there somewhere. It does not require transcendence. To appreciate it you must have both feet firmly on the ground and be anchored firmly in your body—the same way you practice Intuitive Eating and mindfulness. Only from that place of embodied presence can you experience true reverence, satisfaction, contentment, and beauty. Magic.

MINDFUL MOMENT: Notice Everyday Magic

Grab your journal but know this isn't just an exercise to do now. This is a practice I suggest you bring into your everyday life.

Consider how often you notice, appreciate, and express gratitude for what you do have, for the little things, for the tiniest glimpses of beauty, tenderness, and humanity. If you do this often, what conditions allow you to notice? If you don't do this often, what gets in the way?

At the end of each day, try to recall three moments of ordinary, everyday magic: the leaf spiraling to the ground, spontaneous laughter during your kid's bath time, that first delightful sip of coffee. Try to discern what conditions make it easier and harder for you to notice these instances.

Drawing on your evolving understanding of mindfulness of body, mindfulness of feeling, and mindfulness of mind, consider what it might look and feel like to bring the openness, attunement, and resilience of mindfulness and Intuitive Eating into other important aspects of your life. In your journal, please explore any subjects missing from this list and feel free to reach out and share your story! I look forward to hearing from you.

What Can You Celebrate?

- How has noticing your relationship with food and your body reflected on your life?

- What other aspects of your life have been influenced by respecting your inner wisdom?

- Where would you like to bring greater awareness, compassion, or openness into your everyday life?

CHAPTER 14

The Power of Showing Up

Remember those four noble truths?

1. The truth of suffering

2. The cause of suffering

3. The cessation of suffering

4. The path to the cessation of suffering

Recall, the first noble truth does not mean all of life is suffering. Only that parts of life are difficult and this is not something you can escape. Emotional and physical pain, disappointment, change, and loss—from the tiniest discomforts to the grandest agonies, the suffering of life is simply a reality of being born human. That can be difficult to accept.

Our culture teaches us that suffering is optional. That if something doesn't feel good to you, you need to change it, pronto. If you don't, you're doing something wrong. By all means, if something is causing you pain and you can alleviate that pain without harming yourself or anyone else, please do it. But what about when avoiding suffering is not possible?

When suffering is out of your control, you are faced with a decision: figure out how to deal with reality, or try to dodge it. The second noble truth highlights how the dodge actually leads to more suffering: the suffering of suffering. Now that you have this information, what will you do with it?

By now I hope you can have compassion for yourself and your natural aversion to suffering. I hope you can understand the connections between dysfunctional thoughts and behaviors around food, body, and weight and your desire to feel safe. I hope you are gradually becoming a little more comfortable with discomfort. Because there will be a lot of it throughout your life, and knowing you are equipped to deal with it can make that reality a little easier to navigate.

Intuitive Eating and mindfulness form a foundation that supports you to navigate life: your real life, which includes some unavoidable suffering. By tending to your body's needs in a way that creates resilience, stability, and flexibility. By attuning to your emotions so you can truly feel them, understand them, and respond to them. And inevitably by learning to tolerate and expand to accommodate some of the suffering of being human.

Everything changes. Our bodies go through illness and injuries, life stages, aging, and ultimately death. Our priorities and values continue to evolve. Our schedules and environments are constantly shifting, requiring that we adapt again and again. As we move through these changes, the best we can do is notice, feel, adjust, and experiment with new ways of caring for ourselves.

In nurturing your Intuitive Eating practice, keep coming back. Assess how you are working with its elements—hunger, fullness, satisfaction, movement, emotions, mind-set—and recommit and reengage as necessary. Emphasize the constancy of your attention to your overall Intuitive Eating practice instead of judging yourself for not being perfectly consistent in every aspect.

The fourth noble truth defines a path to the cessation of suffering. Lean on your mindfulness and meditation practices to navigate difficult times. Even if months have gone by, find five minutes to sit. Find your posture. Notice what happens when you take your seat—when you root down through the sitz bones and lift up gently through the crown of the head. Acknowledge the dignity of your body and the fierceness in sitting up tall in the midst of this crazy world to feel—to truly feel. There is power in this willingness to feel, allow, and be with yourself. There is power in showing up.

Ironically, the willingness to feel discomfort gives you access to joy, delight, and ecstasy. In protecting yourself from suffering, you also blunt your experience of happiness and pleasure. In opening to your full life, you can feel it all. And this is how to live a life of meaning, depth, and richness.

Imagine if everyone could tolerate their own suffering rather than internalizing it and making themselves into problems or discharging it in ways that harm themselves or others. Imagine if suffering could be regarded as an important element of our experience, one that teaches us what we need to learn and connects us with others through compassion and empathy. Imagine if, through that connection, we could collaborate to solve both individual and collective problems.

It all begins with a breath. A full, deep, completely present breath in your intelligent body is the beginning, middle, and end of this practice.

MINDFUL MOMENT: One Breath

Take a seat or lie down. You can do this practice any time in your waking and walking-about life. Simply stop what you are doing, place your hand over your heart, and take one deep, long, embodied breath. Feel the air becoming breath as it enters your nose and fills your lungs. Feel the breath becoming air as it dissolves back into the space around you. In that moment, in that breath, you are here right now. You are at home in your body. Living your real life. This practice is always available to you. Repeat as necessary.

Conclusion

My own path to self-acceptance has been bumpy: fears, anxiety, depression, existential crises, more anxiety, dieting, addiction, therapy, meditation, and Intuitive Eating. Each of these overlapping phases has been difficult but, more importantly, they have made me who I am now and who I'm becoming.

The philosophy inherent in both Intuitive Eating and mindfulness has shifted my perspective to one of gratitude, even—maybe especially—for my struggles. Without them, I could never understand the heartbreaking reality of being human. I couldn't offer real compassion to my clients. What I have learned during that awkward moment between birth and death is there is nothing wrong with me. There never was. Not that I couldn't continue to learn and become more skillful about navigating life. But at the core, I am okay.

I see a similar struggle play out with each of my clients. Some version of figuring out whether they are okay as they grapple with questions of identity, gender, sexuality, desire, relationships, aging, success, and their ever-changing bodies and how they care for them. They are working through issues around trauma, racism, sexism, mental illness, physical illness, emotions repressed and untended to, unmet needs, inequities. And they are just trying to feel safe.

I have seen the practice of Intuitive Eating, when coupled with mindfulness, give these incredibly capable, talented, sensitive, compassionate individuals glimpses of freedom. Freedom from the prison of thinking they are problems to be solved. The practices of Intuitive Eating and meditation show them again and again that their bodies are good, their hearts are pure, their minds are sharp and trustworthy. We all deserve that. You deserve that.

The curious paradox for me (in addition to that described by Carl Rogers in chapter 1) is the more I have focused on my physical body—its pain, pleasure, sensations, satisfaction, and movement—the more I have felt drawn toward others and the world. The more I care for myself, the more I wish to care for friends, family, clients, and community. The more I tend to my physical and emotional needs, the more motivated I am to address injustices like racism, sexism, ableism, classism, ageism, fatphobia, transphobia—all of the -isms and -phobias.

This makes me wonder what the world would be like if we could all access these teachings. If we worked *with* rather than against our bodies. If we could live with the embodied knowledge of our goodness, wholeness, worthiness. All bodies are inherently worthy. There is nothing wrong with us. We are the experts of ourselves. When we know this, we are powerful.

We can get there. It begins with how we treat our bodies. How you treat your body. Paying attention. Noticing. Feeling. Appreciating. Working with. Speaking to yourself with kindness and compassion. Trusting the process and your intelligent self.

Now that you've completed the book, you have options. You could put it down, take a deep breath, and live your life with attention to feeling and noticing your body, mind, and heart. You could turn back to a chapter or section that felt compelling and take a deeper dive. You could come back to the Intuitive Eating book or workbook and repeat some of the exercises with mindful attention.

Whatever you choose, begin by identifying what has become more natural for you. What is going well? How are you caring for yourself? What are you noticing? Now celebrate yourself. Celebrate how the time, effort, and attention you have directed toward yourself has come to fruition. Celebrate how your continued efforts are planting seeds that will blossom in their own time. Please do not forget to celebrate, even if it is simply that you can notice something you couldn't before.

You can do this. I'm rooting for you. All Intuitive Eaters are.

Acknowledgments

To my clients, who inspire me every day with their intelligence, humor, vulnerability, and compassion. To Evelyn Tribole, MS, RDN, CEDRD-S; Elyse Resch, MS, RDN, CEDRD-S, FAND; and Tracy Tylka, PhD, for sharing these concepts and practices with all of us. To my teachers, Susan Piver, Pema Chödrön, and Chögyam Trungpa, for their guidance in working with things as they are, fiercely and compassionately. To Lisa Fehl, for always being there and imagining the best. To my editors, Ryan Buresh and Jennifer Holder, for understanding this vision and holding me to the highest standards. To Karen Levy, for being just the stickler I needed. To the communities supporting true body liberation: the Intuitive Eating community, the Health at Every Size community, the Association for Size Diversity and Health (ASDAH), Weight-Inclusive Nutrition & Dietetics (WIND), the International Federation of Eating Disorder Dietitians (IFEDD), and the Embodied Social Justice community—you are the future. To my RD Peer Supervision Posse, Robin Millet, MS, RD, CEDRD, CDN; Monika Saigal, MS, RD, CEDRD-S; Justine Roth, MS, CEDRD; and Mary Jane Detroyer, RDN, for keeping me sane during COVID. To Terry Hollenstein and Peter Hollenstein, for always supporting my work and me. And to my partner, Andrea Ventura, and my son, Mimmo: you are my delights! You can have me back now.

Notes

1. Carl Rogers, *On Becoming a Person: A Therapist's View of Psychotherapy*, (New York: Houghton Mifflin Harcourt, 1961).

2. B. K. Hölzel, J. Carmody, M. Vangel, et al., "Mindfulness Practice Leads to Increases in Regional Brain Gray Matter Density," *Psychiatry Research* 191, no. 1 (2011): 36–43.

3. J. Gibson, "Mindfulness, Interoception, and the Body: A Contemporary Perspective," *Frontiers in Psychology* 10 (2019): 2012.

4. Y. Ooishi, M. Fujino, V. Inoue, M. Nomura, and N. Kitagawa, "Differential Effects of Focused Attention and Open Monitoring Meditation on Autonomic Cardiac Modulation and Cortisol Secretion," *Frontiers in Physiology* 12 (2021): 675899.

5. J. Wielgosz, S. B. Goldberg, T. R. A. Kral, J. D. Dunne, and R. J. Davidson, "Mindfulness Meditation and Psychopathology," *Annual Review of Clinical Psychology* 15 (2019): 285–316.

6. D. P. Lippelt, B. Hommel, and L. S. Colzato, "Focused Attention, Open Monitoring and Loving Kindness Meditation: Effects on Attention, Conflict Monitoring, and Creativity—A Review," *Frontiers in Psychology* 5 (2014): 1083.

7. D. Laneri, S. Krach, F. M. Paulus, et al., "Mindfulness Meditation Regulates Anterior Insula Activity During Empathy for Social Pain," *Human Brain Mapping* 38, no. 8 (2017): 4034–46.

8. Jon Kabat-Zinn, "Too Early to Tell: The Potential Impact and Challenges—Ethical and Otherwise—Inherent in the Mainstreaming of Dharma in an Increasingly Dystopian World," *Mindfulness* 8, no. 5 (2017): 1125–35.

9. D. Krishnakumar, M. R. Hamblin, and S. Lakshmanan, "Meditation and Yoga Can Modulate Brain Mechanisms That Affect Behavior and Anxiety—A Modern Scientific Perspective," *Ancient Science* 2, no. 1 (2015): 13–19.

10. T. Gard, M. Taquet, R. Dixit, et al., "Fluid Intelligence and Brain Functional Organization in Aging Yoga and Meditation Practitioners," *Frontiers in Aging Neuroscience* 6 (2014): 76.

11. S. W. Porges, "The Polyvagal Theory: New Insights into Adaptive Reactions of the Autonomic Nervous System," *Cleveland Clinic Journal of Medicine* 76, Supplement 2 (2009): S86–S90.

12. I. Amihai and M. Kozhevnikov, "The Influence of Buddhist Meditation Traditions on the Autonomic System and Attention," *BioMed Research International* 2 (2015): 1–13.

13. T. Pinna and D. J. Edwards, "A Systematic Review of Associations Between Interoception, Vagal Tone, and Emotional Regulation: Potential Applications for Mental Health, Wellbeing, Psychological Flexibility, and Chronic Conditions," *Frontiers in Psychology* 11 (2020): 1792.

14. C. P. Herman and D. Mack, "Restrained and Unrestrained Eating," *Journal of Personality* 43, no. 4 (1975): 647–60.

15. A. R. Lucas, H. D. Klepin, S. W. Porges, and W. J. Rejeski, "Mindfulness-Based Movement: A Polyvagal Perspective," *Integrative Cancer Therapies* 17, no. 1 (2018): 5–15.

16. K. Nay, W. J. Smiles, J. Kaiser, et al., "Molecular Mechanisms Underlying the Beneficial Effects of Exercise on Brain Function and Neurological Disorders," *International Journal of Molecular Sciences* 22, no. 8 (2021): 4052.

17. N. T. van Dam, M. K. van Vugt, D. R. Vago, et al., "Mind the Hype: A Critical Evaluation and Prescriptive Agenda for Research on Mindfulness and Meditation," *Perspectives on Psychological Science* 13, no. 1 (2018): 36–61.

18. L. Nummenmaa, R. Hari, J. K. Hietanen, and E. Glerean, "Maps of Subjective Feelings," *Proceedings of the National Academy of Sciences* 115, no. 37 (2018): 9198–9203.

19. M. R. Tolahunase, R. Sagar, M. Faiq, and R. Dada, "Yoga- and Meditation-Based Lifestyle Intervention Increases Neuroplasticity and Reduces Severity of Major Depressive Disorder: A Randomized Controlled Trial," *Restorative Neurology and Neuroscience* 36, no. 3 (2018): 423–42.

20. The Work of Byron Katie, https://thework.com/instruction-the-work-byron-katie (accessed February 15, 2022).

21. E. R. Albertson, K. D. Neff, and K. E. Dill-Shackleford, "Self-Compassion and Body Dissatisfaction in Women: A Randomized Controlled Trial of a Brief Meditation Intervention," *Mindfulness* 6 (2015): 444–54.

Jenna Hollenstein, MS, RD, CDN, is a nutrition therapist, meditation teacher, and author of five books. Her work combines intuitive eating, trauma-sensitive mindfulness, polyvagal theory, and other embodied modalities. Her work has been featured in *Forbes*, *The Wall Street Journal*, *Self*, *Health*, *Lion's Roar*, *Mindful*, *Vogue*, *Elle*, *Glamour*, *Women's World*, and *U.S. News & World Report*. Jenna lives in the greater New York City, NY, area.

Real change *is* possible

For more than forty-five years, New Harbinger has published proven-effective self-help books and pioneering workbooks to help readers of all ages and backgrounds improve mental health and well-being, and achieve lasting personal growth. In addition, our spirituality books offer profound guidance for deepening awareness and cultivating healing, self-discovery, and fulfillment.

Founded by psychologist Matthew McKay and Patrick Fanning, New Harbinger is proud to be an independent, employee-owned company. Our books reflect our core values of integrity, innovation, commitment, sustainability, compassion, and trust. Written by leaders in the field and recommended by therapists worldwide, New Harbinger books are practical, accessible, and provide real tools for real change.

 newharbingerpublications

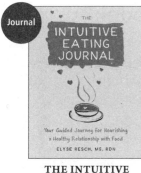
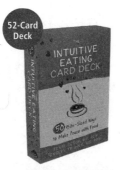
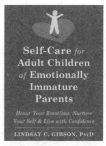
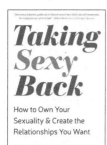
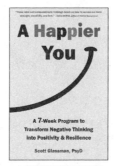
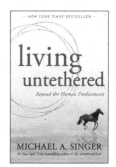

Did you know there are **free tools** you can download for this book?

Free tools are things like **worksheets, guided meditation exercises**, and **more** that will help you get the most out of your book.

You can download free tools for this book—whether you bought or borrowed it, in any format, from any source—from the New Harbinger website. All you need is a NewHarbinger.com account. Just use the URL provided in this book to view the free tools that are available for it. Then, click on the "download" button for the free tool you want, and follow the prompts that appear to log in to your NewHarbinger.com account and download the material.

You can also save the free tools for this book to your **Free Tools Library** so you can access them again anytime, just by logging in to your account! Just look for this button on the book's free tools page.

+ Save this to my free tools library

If you need help accessing or downloading free tools, visit **newharbinger.com/faq** or contact us at **customerservice@newharbinger.com**.